BIG HAIR

BIG HAIR

A JOURNEY INTO THE TRANSFORMATION OF SELF

GRANT McCRACKEN

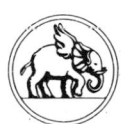

THE OVERLOOK PRESS
WOODSTOCK · NEW YORK

First published in the United States in 1996 by
The Overlook Press
Lewis Hollow Road
Woodstock, New York 12498

Library of Congress Cataloging-in-Publication Data

McCracken, Grant David, 1951-
Big hair : a journey into the transformation of self /
Grant McCracken.
p. cm.
1. Hairdressing–Social aspects. 2. Hairstyles–Social aspects.
I. Title.
GT2290.M354 1996
391'.5—dc20
95-47536
CIP
Originally published by the Penguin Group
Photograph credits on page 217
In order to protect the privacy of people who appear in this
book, their names, in some cases, have been changed
ISBN: 0-87951-657-7
Manufactured in the United States of America
First American Edition

To the memory of my grandmothers,
Shirley Barnhardt Brewer Smith
and Annie Eliza Matthews

Acknowledgments

Thanks are due to many interviewees, readers, friends, colleagues and inspirations: Lynn Appleby, Jane Ayre, Ulana Baluk, Catharine Barnes, Ronnie Burbank, Jeanette Burnside, Barb Campbell, Marjorie Chan, Hsiufen Chou, Carolyn Chow, Ray Civello, Howard Collinson, Chris Commins, Virginia Cooper, Karen Cossar, Carol Costello, Brenda Cowan, Pat Crane, Michael Decsi, Suzanne Deuel, Laima Dingwall, Nicole Eaton, Martha Espenshade, Tim Falconer, Greta Ferguson, Jill Fields, Melanie Fraser, Pat Garner, Judy Globerman, Ron Goldman, Eddie Goodman, Lisa Grant, Robert Gray, Amy Grgich, Lisa Hilderley, Mildred Istona, Jean Jacques Itiera-Alexandre, Basil Johnson, Russell Johnson, Katherine Kay, Naomi Knapp, Anne Lambert, Robert Larkin, Brigitte Laurent, Lori Ledingham, Brenda Lee, Lisa Leibfried, Simon Leung, Anne Lewison, Amy Loewen, Susanne Loewen, Peter Lord, Trisse Loxley, Laurie Ann MacDonald, Emmet McCusker, Helen McLean, Catherine Marjoribanks, Margaret Mark, Julia Matthews, Jessica Miller, Sarah Milroy, Don Mitchell, Erin Mulvey, Brian Musselwhite, Barbara Neckerauer, Judy Nisenholt, Toni Olshen, Punpen Pattarakietiong, Stephen Petrie, Mary Plouffe, Cecelia Potter, John Prevost, Angela Raljic, Rita Rayman, Renata Ambrozio Ribeiro, June Rilett, Linda Scott, Ian Ser, Ping Silvia Shieh, Florence Silver, Lee Simpson, Melodie Smith, David Snell, Ricardo Solera, Monty

Sommers, Diana Stinson, Bob Summers, Marilyn Tan, Guy Thomas, Joan Thompson, Roger Thompson, Liz Torlée, Jamie Tripp, Derek Forbes Waddell, Shannon Sé-am-mé-yeh Wadsworth, Wentworth Walker, Corry Watts, Steve Weiss, Margot Welch, Gene Wilburn, Laena Marie Wilder, Donna Woolcott and Khalil Younes.

Special thanks are due to Jeff Brown, Susan Pointe and Laura Shintani for their superb library, archival and photographic searches; to Jeff Brown, particularly, for putting his exceptional knowledge of Hollywood at my disposal; to Jackie Kaiser, my editor at Penguin, and my agent, Beverley Slopen, for believing in the project when several (male) publishers could not see the point of it; to the Royal Ontario Museum and its director, Dr. John McNeill, for giving me the leave during which this book was researched and written; to Jim Dingwall and Alan Middleton, my colleagues at large, for inspiration and drinks Friday noon; to Adrienne Hood and Trudy Nicks, my colleagues at the museum, for inspiration and drinks Tuesday nights! And first and last, thanks to my sister, Syd McCusker, for the title and the starting point.

This book could not have been written without the contributions of many people. I am hoping readers will contribute to this study of hair by writing with comments, observations and, most important, stories from their own experience. I can be reached at the Royal Ontario Museum, where my address is Department of Ethnology, 100 Queen's Park, Toronto, ON, M5S 2C6. Please do write!

Contents

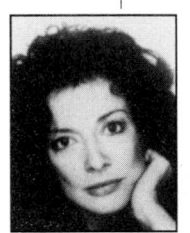

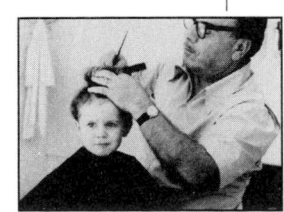

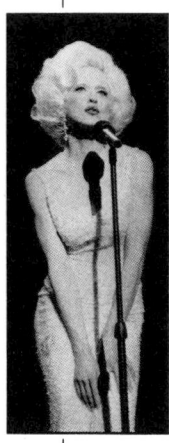
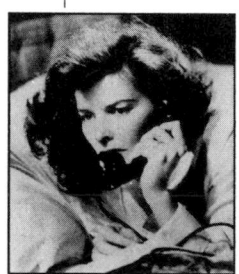

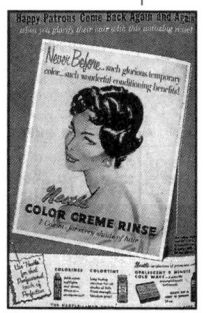
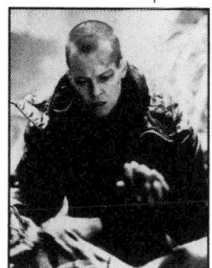

Big

Hair

*unless you grasp
the significance of hair,
you cannot know
the power instilled in it.*

Don King, 1990

Entering the World of Hair

*T*his is a book about hair: hairstyles, hair colour, hairdressers, hair stories and hair history. It's about the famous people who have changed the way we think about hair, including Vidal Sassoon, Marilyn Monroe, Madonna, Candice Bergen and Linda Evangelista. It's about the hairdressers who rule the world of hair, both the courtly professionals and the bad-mannered tyrants. But mostly, this is a book about women and the astonishing purpose they have found for their hair.

We live in a society that believes, generally, that hair is a trivial matter, a thing of no account, a reflection of female vanity. This book takes another point of view. It seeks to show that hair is one of the imperatives of contemporary life. Hair matters in our culture because it is a way, perhaps the most important way, women transform themselves. And this is what the book is really about: hair as the matter and the method of our self-invention.

This is where I ended up after eighteen months of research. But it's not where I started. In fact, I didn't start at all. The topic took me by surprise. I was out for a drive with my sister, while on a visit home to Vancouver. She was amusing herself, as she likes to do, by commenting on people we passed in the street. Today the theme was hair, and she was being, well, a little mean. She remarked a couple of times on something called "big hair." And she then turned her guns on "bad hair." ("Lady, with hair like that you probably qualify for disaster relief.")

I listened to this with half an ear, as brothers do. And then the anthropologist in me snapped to attention. What was my sister talking about? Why did these words sound so strange to my ears? "What," I found myself wondering, "is big hair? What is bad hair?"

Once I started looking into these mysteries, it become clear that hair was, from an academic point of view, terra incognita. Social scientists have ignored it almost completely. Despite the fact that hair is one of the great preoccupations of contemporary life, that we North Americans spend sixteen billion dollars a year on it, that people will drive two hundred miles through a snowstorm to see their hairdressers, no one has really bothered to look at it.

As the research went forward, I began to see just how peculiar this neglect is. The study of hair, I found out, does *not* take you to the superficial edge of our society, the place where everything silly and insubstantial must dwell. It takes you, instead, to the centre of things. We care about hair because it is one of the ways, sometimes the most important way, women contend with the dizzying complexities of everyday life. It is one of the ways they negotiate the endless succession of changes that make up even the most tranquil of contemporary lives: the career shifts, marriages, births, divorces, retirements. Quietly and unexpectedly, hair has become our court of deliberation, the place where we contemplate who and what we are.

We all now live lives of active transformation. This is one of the great accomplishments of our cultural tradition and one of the great joys of our personal lives. We change often, and a lot. Increasingly, transformation has become the single constant of our lives.

These changes are astonishing. We can go from being a person who cares passionately about her social life to someone who wants nothing more than a solitary walk in the country, spaniel in tow. From someone who never misses the Sunday *Times* to someone who hardly ever reads the local paper. From someone defined by her children to someone defined by her work. From someone who lives to be married to someone who lives to be single again. In most cultures, any one of these changes would be the work of a lifetime. In our culture, they all occur in a single lifetime … or even in a couple of years.

There was a time when this self-invention was impossible. We were defined by others. Religion, the community, work, in-laws, husbands, children, our ethnic group, our neighbours all were happy to tell us who we were and what to do. Our marching orders came, indeed, from everyone but us. Happily, all these voices have fallen (or are falling) silent. And this is how it should be. Increasingly, we define ourselves for ourselves by ourselves. More and more, we are free to exercise the right of self-invention.

And now a problem has emerged. How do we deal with this new freedom? There is something thrilling and wonderful about surfing from self to self, about identities that are increasingly labile, fluid, free-floating. But sometimes we find ourselves hankering after the comforting certainties of the traditional agricultural community or a small-town world. From time to time we miss having lives scripted by the verities of a Norman Rockwell portrait.

Certainly, we have all those "self-help" psychologies. But none addresses the real nature of the problem. What we need is *not* better weight control, self-confidence, time management, parenting or back hand (though none of these would hurt). The real, more fundamental problem (and possibility) is that our lives are now a constant succession of selves. We move from one to the next, as if they were so many rocks in the stream. Sometimes passage is easy. Sometimes we slip and fall. In the absence of a formal solution, we have no choice but to keep moving and hope for the best.

The issue is clear enough. Along with our astonishing new freedom, there is a new challenge. We must learn to keep our footing atop the dual circus horses of choice and change. We must learn how to exercise the liberty of self-invention and the new arts of personal transformation. It's time for us to think more systematically and consciously about how we manage our rich and complicated portfolio of selves.

Women have come up with an unofficial answer. Without anyone noticing, they went out and invented their own solution. While all the experts were looking the other way, women found their own instrument for self-transformation. In their hair. This book is about how this happened and what it means. It's about how we use our hair to audition and annex new selves, to seek out new versatility and variety in the people we are, to make our way from rock to slippery rock in the Heraclitean stream of contemporary life. It's about how hairdressers, the good ones anyhow, serve as transformational partners. It's about how haircuts and hair colours have become definitional resources for the constructions of our new, free-floating selves. It's about how hair has become our best instrument of self-invention, our best solution to the problem of constant change. The day is coming when virtual reality and the reworking of DNA will give us new transformational opportunities. But, for the moment, our transformational instrument is our hair.

A word on how I wrote this book is probably in order. After years of indifference, the scholarly world is suddenly producing academic books and articles on the subject of popular culture. (Not on hair, mind you, but movies, television, toys and cars have suddenly become legitimate topics.) Unhappily, much of this work is flawed.

The problem is a simple one. Scholars (especially the ones in the "critical" and the "cultural" schools) have decided they may study the contemporary world without actually talking to anyone who lives inside of it. Several hundred books have been written in the last decade by scholars who have never once left the safety and comfort of an armchair. In this La-Z-Boy anthropology, as I like to call it, the academic never comes in contact with anyone who might contradict his or her intellectually fashionable and politically correct opinions. Thus do scholars preserve the insularity of the university world and, ironically, the inscrutability of the things they presume to study.

Well, anyway, this strikes me as the wrong way to study popular culture. And it is obviously the wrong way to study hair. Clearly, nobody wants a book about what *I* think about hair. This is not just because before I went for that drive with my sister I really had never thought about the topic. Or because I happen to be losing my own hair in a hurry. It's because nobody can get to the bottom of a topic as important and as neglected as this one from the safety and comfort of an armchair. If you want any kind of truth at all, you have to get out and talk to people.

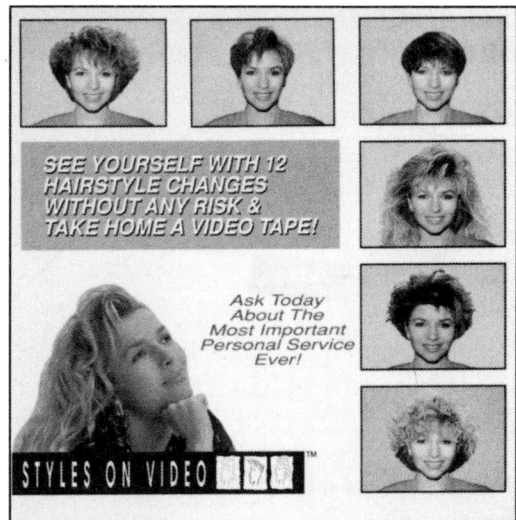

Transformation on video

And I have. I began with one hairdresser, Lawrence, and he introduced me to clients, who introduced me to more hairdressers, who introduced me to more clients, and before long I was chatting with people in Atlanta, Chicago, Dallas, Los Angeles, New York, San Francisco, Seattle, Toronto and Vancouver. Many hours of interviewing. Many cups of coffee. Forests of pens and pencils.

Mountains of paper. Lots and lots of talk.

My contacts sometimes failed me. Then it was necessary to make the "cold call." When I needed to talk to a bouffant, for example, I would screw up my courage and my charm (what there is of it) and stop people on the street. "Hi, I'm doing a study of hair..." Several people thought this was a new pick-up line and just kept walking, but most of them were prepared to slow down and consider the question. "You want to talk to me about my hair?" they would say, their voices ringing with disbelief. "It's for science," I would reassure them piously. "Well, I guess so..." they'd say, and the interview would begin.

There was one group who would not talk to me: men. Lawrence, my ambassador to the world of hair, warned me that this would happen. "Men are much vainer about their hair than women and they're afraid you'll find out! They'll tell you nothing." He was right. After a couple of weeks of trying, I had proof. Men would not participate in the research. Oh, they would sit for the interview, but they'd reveal nothing useful. Apparently, there's a secret rule of masculinity that says, "Hair and style are not guy stuff." As a result, this is, mostly, a book about women's hair. Men, and their hair, appear from time to time, but they are not the first object of our curiosity. Mostly, this book is about women, for women.

Will men be unhappy with this? I don't care if they are. The way I see it, they can't have it both ways. They have declared hair a trivial matter and mocked women for caring about it. They have used hair as a way to control and belittle women. They can't expect to be included when hair is taken seriously.

At the Salon with Cynthia and Bernard

*L*awrence is late. We were supposed to start the interview at ten o'clock, but twenty minutes later there's no sign of him. I'm sitting with my cup of coffee watching the salon gear up for another day. The staff arrive in ones and twos. They look at me with absolutely no curiosity and head straight for the coffee. Someone turns on a radio. You can feel the place starting, reluctantly, to come to life. But still no Lawrence.

The first client arrives. Cynthia is in her late thirties. She's wearing a beautifully tailored teal-blue suit and hauling a large, black briefcase. She has blond hair to her shoulders, a softer version of the Murphy Brown cut. Bernard, her hairdresser, greets her extravagantly and sends her off to the sinks. A few minutes later she returns with her wet hair in a towel. Bernard summons coffee and gets her settled in.

Cynthia's hair is very thick and very blond. Perhaps too blond. Bernard looks like he's contemplating damage control. Cynthia doesn't look very happy either. She is pulling at her hair in fits and starts.

Bernard looks at his client in the mirror and smiles. "What's new, Cynthia?"

"Oh, nothing," she says back to the mirror, "you know, the usual."

"Still busy?"

"I'm so busy I can't see straight," Cynthia says. She sounds tired and a little exasperated.

"That's nice. What's on your wrist?" Bernard is referring to a bandage just above Cynthia's right hand.

Cynthia brightens a little. "Oh, it's a bite. My cat got excited!" She pulls at the bandage and adds, "Doesn't it look terrible? I *would* have to keep playing with it."

Bernard starts playing with an imaginary bandage on his own wrist and says, "Wow, is this ever neat!" And he bats it again, "Hey, this is fun."

There is a sound of someone pounding up the stairs. It's Lawrence. He charges into the salon, apologizes for being late and promises to return after an "essential" phone call. You can see a colossal shiner on his left eye.

The bruise does not escape Cynthia. As Lawrence passes, she bats her eyelashes and asks with comic-opera coyness, "Too much

Cynthia's hair is very thick and very blond

fun last night, Lawrence?" Lawrence pretends he does not hear and keeps on walking. As he passes my chair, he discreetly rolls his eyes.

Cynthia looks at Bernard in the mirror and they smirk simultaneously.

"Kids! You gotta watch 'em every second," Bernard exclaims, and they both laugh out loud.

Someone turns up the radio. Bernard says, "Oh, God, not this again." And then loudly, for the salon to hear, "Do you think we could play something decent for a change, please?"

"My dad's acting kinda strange," Cynthia says abruptly.

"Got the grumpies again?"

"This time it's a new girlfriend."

"Oooo."

"He's never home. He doesn't call. I never see him."

"That's a new girlfriend for you."

"Yeah, but who is this Beverley? I haven't met her. I

haven't even *seen* her."

Bernard says nothing. He is combing out Cynthia's hair in long, systematic strokes.

"I should know something about her. I mean, he doesn't need my approval, obviously. But I should ... I should ..." Cynthia grinds to a halt.

"Check her out," Bernard puts in.

"That's right."

"Get the scoop."

"Exactly," Cynthia says with relief. "Shouldn't I ...?" She trails off again.

"Absolutely. Parents! You gotta watch 'em every second."

Cynthia laughs with relief. "Exactly. Especially him."

"Don't you have your annual meeting coming up?" Bernard asks. "Minneapolis or something?"

"No, Milwaukee."

"You hate Milwaukee."

"I was *born* in Milwaukee."

Bernard mugs her distaste and they both laugh.

"Well, then, what are we going to do with this hair?" he asks.

"I don't like it, Bernard!" Cynthia wails.

Bernard looks thoughtfully at her hair. He is combing it through and watching it fall.

"Any ideas?" she demands.

"We could go shorter," Bernard says in a musing tone.

"Yes, but ..."

"Lots of people are," Bernard says, still musing.

"I'm not a short-hair person. Everything looks like hell on me. Anyway, I'm too young for short hair."

"That's true, that's true," Bernard says in a hurry.

There is a long pause. They are looking at one another in the mirror. Cynthia is miserable. Bernard is still thoughtful.

"How about a new colour?" he asks.

"Like what?" Cynthia is pouting a little.

"Something auburn?" Bernard says tentatively.

"Brown hair!" Cynthia explodes. "Bernard, how long have you known me? I'm a blonde."

Bernard arches his eyebrows and ducks his chin at her in the mirror.

"Okay, not a blonde of nature but a blonde of the spirit. Everyone says so. You say so."

"How about a darker blond? A little less bombshell. Still sunny, but a little less, you know, *ba boom.*"

> *"So what's the approach?" Lawrence asks mockingly. "The big exposé? Dangerous chemicals and slave wages? Hairdressing: the gay profession?"*

"What are you talking about, Bernard? Do you mean *vavoom?*"

"Sorry, that is what I mean. Something less *vavoom.*"

There is a pause as Cynthia thinks about this.

"Me?"

"You. Bright but not bombshell. Warm but not searing. You know, sexual but not siren."

"Me?"

"Absolutely. You, you, you. It's you, Cynthia. Trust me."

Lawrence is still busy with something. By this time, the waiting area has filled up. I'm sitting between two women who are waiting to have their hair done. The one with the blunt cut looks exhausted but content. She has found her refuge. The other wears her hair very short and chic. She's paging through *Vogue* and she stops from time to time to regard herself coolly in the mirror opposite. I can't tell what she thinks of what she sees.

A languid young man is walking around the lobby with a glass atomizer. He is spritzing grandly and declaiming: "I feel energized. The water heals us!"

"Perfuming the air?" I ask as he passes.

He looks at me with indulgence. "I am conditioning it with positive ions."

"Ah," I nod sagely. "Positive ions."

Lawrence comes by to say our interview is next on his list, but first he has to deal with an irate client who hates her perm so much she's threatening legal action. I say I don't mind waiting.

By this time, Bernard has persuaded Cynthia to consider moving away from her bombshell blond to something a little different. She is resisting. She has invested heavily in the blond persona. But somewhere inside her is a small voice of doubt. Something is telling her to move on.

Bernard is pitching the virtues of other kinds of blondness. So far I've counted four variations: "bombshell," which Cynthia is now; "sunny," which Bernard would like her to become; "brassy," which both want to avoid; and "cool," which both agree is completely wrong for her.

"There's one more possibility!" Bernard says.

"What?" Cynthia asks impatiently.

"Donna Mills blond."

"What's that?"

"Kind of 'don't mess with me' blond. Like her old character on 'Knots Landing.' Dangerous ... a little formidable."

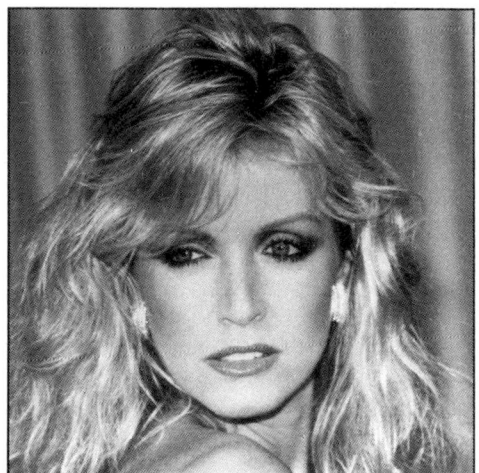

"Could I do that?"

"I think so," Bernard says, thinking about it, and then with more conviction, "Sure you could. The question is, do you want to?"

"I'll tell you what. I'm tired of men getting the wrong idea. I'm tired of morons. Dangerous might be good."

Donna Mills: Dangerous Blond

"I'm not saying it's for you. Sunny is good. Donna Mills is good. For that matter, society blond would be good."

"What's that, like ash blond?"

"Yeah, old-money blond. Kind of glints. You know, polish."

"Was that Polish, Bernard?" Cynthia asks with a look of mischief.

"No, *polish*!" Bernard returns with feeling.

"Bernard, get a grip. That's for rich housewives in their sixties. I'm young. I'm single. And I'm professional." She gives him a "you've got rocks in your head" look.

"So you are. Fair enough. Okay."

Lawrence really does have a shiner, the kind that hurts to look at. He sits down heavily. He's looking a little beleaguered. "I'm sorry," he tells me, shaking his head, "some days come undone earlier than others. This one did so sometime last night. Do you want some more coffee?"

"No, I'm okay." I say, surveying the controlled chaos on all sides of us. "You're busy!"

"You should be here at closing time. So Janet says you're writing a book"—his voice registers a little scepticism—"about hair?"

"I'm scouting the topic."

The "positive ion" guy makes a languid pass with the atomizer. Lawrence gives the kid the papal nod. This is, apparently, the sort of thing he endures routinely from junior staff.

Cynthia passes us. She is being followed by someone who has a handful of what look like little cellophane squares. Cynthia's made her choice, and I missed it. She's getting her hair coloured and I have no idea if she's going to bombshell, sunny or dangerous. Damn.

"So what's the approach?" Lawrence asks mockingly. "The big exposé? Dangerous chemicals and slave wages? Hairdressing: the gay profession?"

"No exposé. No agenda. I want to tell the story from the inside out. To capture the culture of hair. That's it. That's all."

In fact, my objective is simpler. I'd be happy just to understand Cynthia and Bernard. Make sense of that conversation, a little voice tells me, and you can capture the whole world of hair.

A receptionist comes by and bangs Lawrence on the shoulder with her pink message pad.

"That lady is on line one again. She says she's talked to her lawyer and what are you going to do about it."

"Tell her I'm talking to my lawyer and I'll call her back. That should cool her off."

By this time the shop is full and the word is out. Everyone knows the man talking to Lawrence is an anthropologist here to do a book on hair. People are dropping by to listen in. We've drawn a small crowd.

I am, for instance, being scrutinized by a pretty brunette—a colourist, I find out later. She is standing beside Lawrence, listening to every word I say and examining me with a mixture of curiosity and suspicion. I know why she is cautious. When people start talking about hair and hairdressers, the air fills with stereotypes. One is that hairdressers are silly, flighty people. A second is that people who care about hair are silly and flighty. A third is that people care about hair because they have been tricked. (This last idea is enjoying particular currency at the moment. Naomi Wolf, for instance, believes we've been mesmerized by the likes of Clairol, Revlon and L'Oréal.[1])

The colourist is trying to decide whether I am going to pour fuel on this bonfire of misconceptions. Am I one more hit man in the character assassination to which her profession is constantly subjected? Will I implicate her in that millinery-industrial complex that is supposed to conspire against us, turning otherwise sensible people into besotted fools for fashion? She's sceptical. But I have the impression that Lawrence might be coming around.

"So what do you want from me?" he asks.

"Just a chance to talk about hair, as you see it."

"Philosophy—or the nuts and bolts?"

"Whatever you want, preferably both."

Lawrence is fearless. He sits in the middle of this carefully constructed bedlam, with hairdressers, colourists, assistants and apprentices in full motion around him. An interview is just one more demand, one more novelty. There is risk in this interview, but there is risk in virtually everything Lawrence does. He thinks a moment and then he nods.

"Come back Saturday around closing," he almost has to shout over the din. "We'll go for a drink. Someplace quiet."

So begins my expedition into the world of hair.

Five Women in the Works:

Transformations of Self through Style

*A*ny expedition into the world of hair must begin with what we know. And what we "know" about hair is all contained in the book of stereotypes. Hairdressers are flighty, mercurial creatures who like nothing better than to ignore their clients' wishes and impose the latest frivolous fashion. People who care about hair are every bit as bad: they are victims of fashion, captives of vanity, dupes of a marketing conspiracy and happiest when flitting thoughtlessly from look to look. So speak the stereotypes. I ask you to consider the following five stories and decide for yourself.

Cynthia's New Colour

As it turned out, Cynthia followed Bernard's advice and went for "sunny." Reluctantly. I had a chance to talk to her a few days later. Was the new colour a success?

"Maybe I like it, maybe I don't," she said. "I've let that little bastard talk me into new things over the years and it always takes a while to tell. Sometimes he's right. Sometimes he's so wrong I can't believe it. It's wait and see."

Cynthia likes her hair relatively big and very blond. Moving away from bombshell blondness was a risk. She had no idea how people would react. And, more to the point, she had no idea how she would feel. Bombshell was like an old friend. She didn't want to give it up.

Cynthia likes bombshell because she went to private school. It was her idea of rebellion: "Everyone was being so terribly sophisticated. And I thought, the hell with you guys. I didn't want to hide my light under a bushel. I wasn't going to be your goody-two-shoes, the shrinking violet type. I tell you, that school was a training ground for mousy women. The really courageous ones became kindergarten teachers. Nothing wrong with that, but it's not for me, thank you very much."

For Cynthia, bombshell blondness was like turning up the volume on the stereo. She wanted the world to notice her, and when she coloured her hair bright blond, it did. The trouble with this colour, according to Cynthia, was that it sent the wrong kind of signal to the wrong kind of man. With her hair at top volume, she was constantly getting a little too much attention from the construction worker at the corner and her colleagues at work: "They all seem to think I want them to make a fuss. And sometimes it *is* sort of sweet. But, more and more, it feels like they are reacting to my hair, not to me. It feels like it has absolutely nothing to do with me. I want to say 'Get a life.'"

Bernard understands Cynthia well. "Cynthia's the kind of woman who wears her hair like a flag. It's her declaration of independence. She doesn't want to get pegged as Daddy's little rich girl or Lady Gracious. She's an 'in-your-face' type. She wants her hair big and blond. At least, she used to ..."

It was easy for Bernard to see the crisis coming. Cynthia was full of listless complaints. She didn't like the way her hair broke at the shoulders. She thought the colour was a shade off. She wanted Bernard to come up with a brand new idea, but she also wouldn't budge. All classic symptoms, Bernard told me, of a woman primed for change—and petrified of it: "You could tell she was ready to move on and you didn't need to be a rocket scientist to figure out why. In her circles this haircut has never been in fashion, and the '80s killed it for just about everyone else. Frankly, on a woman like her, it's a little embarrassing."

Bernard began the painstaking work of getting Cynthia ready for the big move. "My job is to pry her fingers off the old look. People are funny. They get caught up in the look. Changing it can be like bomb disposal work. You have to be careful. You're talking about more than a haircut."

Bernard wasn't sure the new colour was going to work. "The new colour is not as big as the old one. Cynthia likes to bowl people over. And she's got the personality for it. That's why bombshell worked so well. We've gone to something more sunny. The trouble is, the new colour has a sweetness I'm afraid she'll hate. Don't get me wrong. Cynthia can do sweet. But I'm pretty sure she doesn't want to."

Bernard has his doubts, but right now "sunny" blondness is the only move he can get her to make. This is, as he points out, a long-term process. "Great haircuts are not discovered. They're created. Usually over many months and many cuts. You try this. You try that. In this business, there's no such thing as 'one size fits all.' You're looking for the cut that captures the person. You're looking for the cut that will pull them along. Plus, Cynthia is changing. She's still figuring out what she wants and who she is. We'll get there. We'll get there."

I kept in touch with Cynthia and Bernard. As it turned out, they gave up on "sunny" almost immediately. As Bernard guessed, it was just a little too cheery for Cynthia. They moved towards "dangerous" blond. "We're engineering it bit by bit," Bernard says. "We started with that bitchy, really self-possessed Donna Mills thing. It was good but too cool, so we had to heat it up. Plus, Mills had a really fierce blunt cut. Too severe for us. Cynthia's hair had to be bigger and softer. We started with Mills and went a little warmer and a little softer. Still a little formidable. But not so bitchy.

Not so hard."

By the eight-month mark, Cynthia was looking distinctly more professional than when I saw her first. Her hair was cooler, the cut was clearer. She looked more business and less bombshell. But you could still hear her personality and her sexuality. On the whole she is pleased. "It's really cut down on the yahoo factor," she told me. "Guys still notice me but they don't carry on quite so much. And I still feel like people see me coming. I walk into a room and I command attention. They know I'm there."

I believe Cynthia and Bernard are doing something more interesting than the stereotypes allow.

Barbara's French Knot

Barbara is a long-time client of Lawrence's. They know one another inside out, and Lawrence has great admiration for her: "She's smart and she's thoughtful. She's good to talk to. Be sure to ask her about her first French knot."

Barbara is in her forties. She has three children, all girls. She has a degree in library science and works as an "information manager" at a large company. We are sitting on the deck behind her house. The two older girls, Katy and Lillith, are traipsing around the yard in their mother's old shoes and dresses. Patricia is sound asleep in the hamper beside us.

We have her photo album open and we are trying to piece together the history of Barbara's hair. Looking at the album is a strange experience for her. "It kind of makes my head swim," she says. There are some looks she recognizes. The images of the little girl with her eager grin and her flying braids come back right away. But some are unfamiliar and embarrassing. Barbara looks at some of her teenage pictures and shakes her head with wonder. "Oh, God, how could I have done anything like that?"

One of Barbara's earliest memories is of having her braids done. Every morning her mother would sit her down and transform her hair from the wilderness of sleep into two tidy rows. This was Barbara's ritual of exit. She never left the house without them.

For Barbara, braiding was an adult mystery. Often, she didn't particularly care how her hair was done, she just wanted to go out and play. But for her mother braiding was a way to lavish a little extra attention on her dear little girl. It was a way to arm her against the perils of the world out there. And it was one of the ways this 1950s family struggled to keep up with the Cleavers, the Andersons and all those other tidy families on TV.

Barbara grew to love the ritual. She would stand facing away from her mother. She had to be still, which meant not reaching out to pet a passing cat or swat a taunting brother. "It was the only time I was still all day," she says.

She teased it high. She ironed it flat.

Barbara remembers the agility of her mother's hands as they pulled her hair into place. She remembers her mother talking into her ear, issuing last instructions, begging her to keep her new shoes clean, whispering secrets. "I can still hear her murmuring in my ear," she says. It was comforting and wonderful to hear this voice behind her. It put the world right. It got her ready for the day.

When she was about nine or ten, Barbara's aunt took her for an "adult" treatment, her first.

> The hairdresser took my hair to the back, wound it around and fastened it in. My hair was way too heavy, but I thought this was the height of glamour. I thought it made me look like Grace Kelly. I was enchanted.

Barbara suddenly saw the point of hair. The braids had never really grabbed her, but this French knot was something else. "It made me feel different. It made me look different. I realized when you do your hair, something can happen." The end of braids was the beginning of something new.

As Barbara entered her teen years, she embarked upon a career of experimentation. She tried out all the looks. She put her hair up. She teased it high. She ironed it flat. She treated it with peroxide, Tonis and Dippity-doo. She even washed it with that great technical advance of the 1960s, "dry shampoo."

She was no longer taking her cue from her mother. Now she consulted a circle of girlfriends. And they consulted endlessly—after school, at pyjama parties and for hours on the phone. Within a few years, Barbara was a master tactician. There was virtually nothing she could not do with her hair. No strategy or artifice was too strange or too hard. Barbara was a virtuoso.

This was not art for its own sake. It was what Barbara calls her ticket to the world of sock hops and the "drive-in" car culture of the '50s and early '60s. Barbara looks back and laughs. "Let's face it. We were hood ornaments. A guy spent a lot of time on his car and he wanted a chick who would look good beside him."

Barbara remembers going through a lot of guys and a lot of hairspray. "We used to kill our hair. It had to be fat, high and really smooth. That took lots of teasing, lots of hairspray and lots of time. The guys spent all their time styling their cars and we spent all our time styling our hair."

But this too passed. Around seventeen, Barbara got caught up in the tremendous cultural change that was taking place. She became a hippie. Suddenly, all the old principles of hair care were forsaken. No more rollers, hairspray or teasing. The very idea of manipulating hair was now out of fashion. In fact, *fashion* was out of fashion. Now the idea was to let hair do its own thing. "We thought hair was beautiful just the way it was."

People were now treating their hair with the same tender regard they showed their feelings. Neither were for cultivation or discipline. You and your hair were supposed to be free. Every strand of hair was supposed to have its own place in the world.

So much for the ideology of hair. But in fact, women still cared about style and they still worked hard at it. And there were several styles to work at. Sometimes Barbara was the Earth Mother, sometimes the Indian Princess, sometimes the LSD Fantasy Queen, sometimes the SDS Revolutionary. These looks were all quite different, but most required headbands.

Barbara's mother hated virtually all these looks:

> My mother used to say, "When are you going to grow up and get your hair cut?" And I recall thinking "This is the real mark of my decline. This is the beginning of the end. I'll get my hair cut and end up just like my mother." I kept thinking, "That's what grownups do, cut their hair, and lead long, boring lives."

The hair her mother had so carefully braided every morning had become a battleground. The issue was clear. "She wanted my hair to match *her* idea of who I was. I wanted it to match *my* idea of who I was. The older I got, the more I felt that my hair should be my decision."

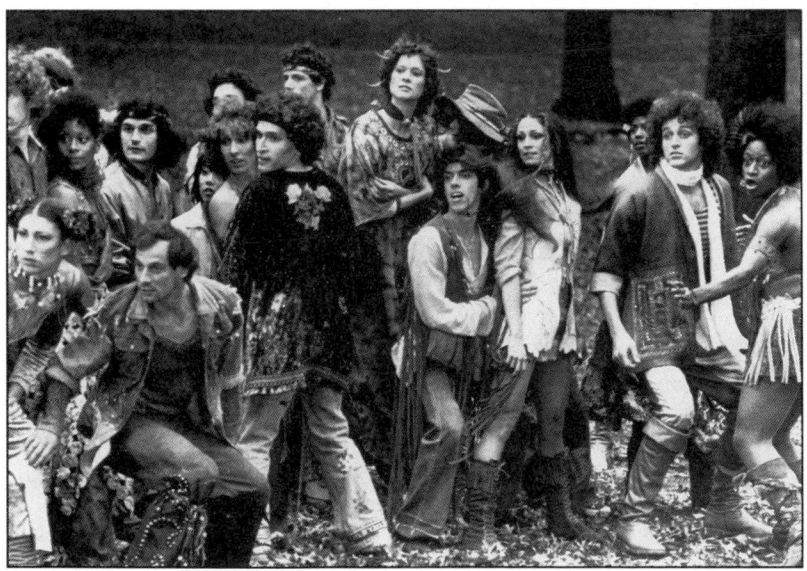

Hair at liberty

A Woman Made Fun Of

Janet is about thirty-six, a homemaker, a mother of two. She doesn't have a career outside the home. Her kids are the centre of her life, and they are wonderful. Though she asked them to stay out of the kitchen while we did the interview in the breakfast nook, every so often they would appear in the doorway to stare at us without a sound, their faces alive with intelligence and character.

But this home has not always been an easy place for Janet. There have been moments in her life, she told me, when she felt it was all too much for her. Or, more accurately, that it was all not nearly enough. She loved her kids and she was obviously a gifted mom, but she could not shake the feeling that things were passing her by. "I guess I needed a change," she says. "I found myself dreaming about being in Greece or Paris. Any place but here. I believed everybody had a more exciting life than me."

There was no easy answer. She wasn't about to up and leave the family. Her kids needed her. Then a friend suggested that she try a new hair colour. "I dyed it myself. I'd always wanted to be a redhead so that's what I became. I remember being so excited. It was wonderful you could make this kind of change. I felt like I was more sophisticated, that I could do things, that we could go out of the house, that the humdrumness was going away. It was amazing."

What was even more amazing was the reaction from other people. Everybody hated the new look. Her husband recoiled, her friends were revolted, and her sisters were openly contemptuous.

Janet was crushed. The hair colour that set her free from domesticity was rejected by just about everyone. A cousin was particularly cruel. Janet tried to defend herself. She said, "Hey, I'm just trying to get with the '90s." The cousin replied, "Try going through the '80s first."

The hostility proved to be more than Janet could bear and she switched back to her natural colour. "I didn't pass the approval test so I didn't pursue it any further." And she is still not sure exactly what happened. She remembers thinking, "They're afraid of what I might become. They need me to remain the way I am."

Lawrence and Ruth

One of Lawrence's most interesting stories is about Ruth. Ruth is on the verge of adolescence, and she has chosen to look like a boy. She wears male clothing and walks a male walk. She has cut her hair very short and covers it, usually, with a baseball hat.

Lawrence saw Ruth on the several occasions she came to the salon to wait for her mother. She would sit in the waiting room with her baseball cap pulled low over her eyes, the picture of unhappiness. Her boyish image was so striking that Lawrence's staff openly speculated that Ruth was on her way to a "radical" gender choice. Ruth's mother was haunted by the same conclusion.

Lawrence could feel the tension between mother and daughter. He decided to intervene and he saw immediately that he had several tasks, the first of which was to calm the mother. In his thoughtful way, Lawrence gave the mother a chance to articulate her anxieties, and then he gently eased them. He told her Ruth was well within the envelope of the normal. Lawrence knew that the mother did not buy this for a second, but he also knew that she was immensely reassured to hear it said.

The second task was to keep himself from getting on the bandwagon:

> I could see the visual. I could see what my staff meant. But I give everybody great capacity for change, to be multi-dimensional. I hate to lock somebody into [an image], because as soon as I do, their haircut is never going to change. I'm going to focus on them one way. I'm not going to allow them to

change. So I might as well stop being their hairdresser right now.

The third challenge was to get Ruth into the chair.
This was the hard part. Naturally, Ruth's mom wanted
nothing more than to submit her daughter to the attentions of her own hairdresser. Just as naturally, Ruth wanted
nothing less.

Lawrence began his campaign. He made a point of
chatting to Ruth while she sat in the waiting area. He made
a point of disagreeing with her mother in a gentle, mocking
way when Ruth was present, to show his independence.

Eventually he prevailed. One day, out of the blue, while
her mom was putting on her coat, Ruth asked for a book-
ing. Her mother was astonished. Lawrence was thrilled: "I
went into the stockroom and did a victory dance."

At first, it was every bit as awkward as Lawrence had
expected. On the one side, a mother privately pleaded
with Lawrence to use his transformational powers to
"save" her daughter. On the other, a cautious, distrustful,
pubescent girl watched his every move, weighed his every
remark. "You could say it went slowly," he recalls.

Lawrence did what every good hairdresser does. He
identified himself with Ruth, slipping into her self, beginning
to see the world as she sees it. And it worked. Ruth came
to see him as a likeable, unthreatening guy, as someone
who looked at her without comment or judgment, as
someone who understood her because he was, finally and
unexpectedly, a lot like her. "We talked music, clothing. We
talked hair," Lawrence says. "I told her I've gone short and
long and everything in between. I can find something in
common with anyone. But it turned out we had a lot in
common anyway."

As they talked, a connection was fashioned. Lawrence
came to understand Ruth and she him. Ruth was not necessarily preparing herself for a lifetime of mannish haircuts.
She was merely in a state of suspension. She was on the

edge of becoming a woman, but she had no real idea how this was to be accomplished or who she wanted to be. She disliked many of the images before her. She found others confusing or conflicting.

"I think this is why some young girls become anorexic," Lawrence says. "Their bodies are rushing towards womanhood and their nerve snaps. They lose their confidence. The best way to put the brakes on is to starve back their womanhood. This is what Ruth was doing with the baseball hats. She was keeping the whole womanhood thing at bay."

Lawrence's ministrations worked well. Before long, Ruth was no longer hiding out in her gender disguise. She was chattering away to Lawrence about her options. All of a sudden she was auditioning selves.

Lawrence doesn't know how the metamorphosis will end. "There is a wonderful young woman here. She's going to be big and tall and beautiful. Maybe she'll stick with baseball caps and crew cuts. It doesn't matter. My job is to see that whatever she does, she does as a choice ... and that she looks great, of course." And then he smiles a beautiful smile of his own. "Whatever Ruth does, it's going to be spectacular."

Brenda and Corporate Hair in the '80s and '90s

Brenda is a lawyer. She works in the offices of a corporate law firm, a vast enterprise that takes up many floors of a downtown office tower. I met her there several years ago. I'm not sure what I was expecting but I was not expecting Brenda. She was tall, big-boned and splendid in a black-and-purple Chanel suit. What was most striking was her helmet of jet-black hair, a blunt cut with lots of volume. This hair framed a strong face and

Brenda was gracious and charming about it but she smoked them

large, handsome blue eyes. Brenda looked like something out of "L.A. Law."

I watched Brenda at work in a series of negotiations. She was facing an opposing lawyer (a woman, like Brenda, in her middle thirties) and a number of administrators, all men. Brenda was formidable and discriminating in her suit and perfect coiffure.

The opposing lawyer and her companions had another look together. One of the men was dressed in a bad suit and museum-quality Beatle boots. Beside him sat the lawyer for the opposition in an elaborately pleated blouse (something like an Elizabethan ruff with the air let out), a long peasant skirt in an African print, Birkenstock sandals and a long, flowing, unstructured haircut.

"L.A. Law" cast

Brenda sat on one side of the negotiating table like an elegant bird of prey who hadn't quite decided where to begin her meal. Her hair and clothing spoke volumes:

> I am a woman of perfect, steadfast professionalism. You can depend upon me to take responsibility for my work and to do it according to the highest professional standard. Let no one (and especially no man) take me lightly or for granted. Let no one underestimate me. What is not defended in the course of these negotiations is mine. What is not nailed down at the end of these negotiations is mine.

Mistakes, errors of judgment, miscalculations on your part all accrue to me. I am, in a good-natured, kind-hearted way, pitiless and inexorable. I will make no mistakes and I will forgive none. I am not cold-blooded, heartless or unfeeling. I am simply professional.

The opposing lawyer's look told another story. It said:

I am no creature of fashion. I am no creature of the market place. I am no cold-hearted individualist. I am no sharpie, no smoothie, no fast-talker, no opportunist. I believe in a kinder, gentler world. I believe in the solidarity of the group over the selfish, grasping ambition of the individual. I am not driven by self-interest. I answer to a higher calling and a broader view. Take this clothing and this hair as a token of my goodwill, my kindness and my compassion. I am, above all, as you can see, a decent person.

As it turned out, Brenda won. She was gracious and charming about it but she smoked them. I have never thought about the phrase "high-powered lawyer" quite the same way since.

Brenda's blunt cut was a signature symbol for the 1980s. It did for women's hair what the "dress for success" look did for women's clothing. It refused the conventional symbolism. It refused anything that was undisciplined, poetic, free-flowing, romantic, sensual or evocative.

There are, of course, many ways a woman can be attractive. She can be "pretty," "lovely," "winsome," "cute," "gorgeous" or "beautiful."

After all, women had displayed these qualities only to have them used against them, as proof that they could not be taken seriously in the world of work, that they could not be trusted with real responsibility. The blunt cut exploded the gilded cage that imprisoned women in the role of gentle, bending creatures. It created a new message, a new symbolism for women. It said: "What is true of

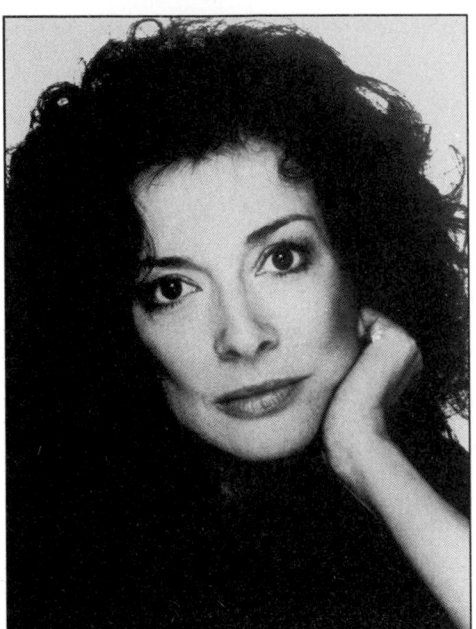

Dixie Carter: Handsome Hair

the hair is true of the woman; both are perfectly balanced, disciplined, controlled and professional."

Brenda's hair had a second layer of symbolism. Nature (or her hairdresser) had made it a striking black. This had a message, too: "I am what you see before you, a creature of stark contrast, a woman who does not admit to shades of grey, giddy blondness or flamboyant red. I will not be a prisoner of your sexist expectations. I am not an accommodating, adaptable, flexible female. I am uncompromising."

There was a third layer of symbolism. Brenda's blunt cut had depth. This too sent a message. In contrast to the wispy haircut of the opposing lawyer, this cut said: "I am substantial, I am unmistakable. Overlook me at your peril."

The fourth layer of symbolism was the best one of all. The cut was calculated to make Brenda *handsome*. There are, of course, many ways a woman can be attractive. She can be "pretty," "lovely," "winsome," "cute," "gorgeous" or "beautiful." In the professional world, however, each of these terms of praise can have a disadvantage. A sexist colleague might suppose (or merely claim) that she is not fully qualified. ("Aren't you a pretty little thing. Don't tell me you type, too?")

It's hard to dismiss or diminish "handsome" in this way. Handsome is attractive without the down-side. Handsome women have stature, grace and presence.

(Dixie Carter on TV's "Designing Women" is a good case in point; Diane Sawyer is another.) There is nothing diminutive or decorative about them. In all of this, Brenda knew exactly what she was doing. She was making "Brenda."

Brenda's Search for '90s Hair

Things have changed. Brenda's blunt cut was, like the Chanel suit, the perfect look for the 1980s. And both are beginning to pass from fashion. As Holly Brubach put it recently in the pages of *The New Yorker*, "The Chanel suit, the uniform of the eighties, with its combined message of career, money and sex, is losing its totemic powers. Already its glamour has begun to seem quaint ...."[1] This applies equally to the blunt cut. Its moment, too, is beginning to pass.

Trouble is, of course, we're not quite clear what the new decade is. Some claim the '90s are less competitive,

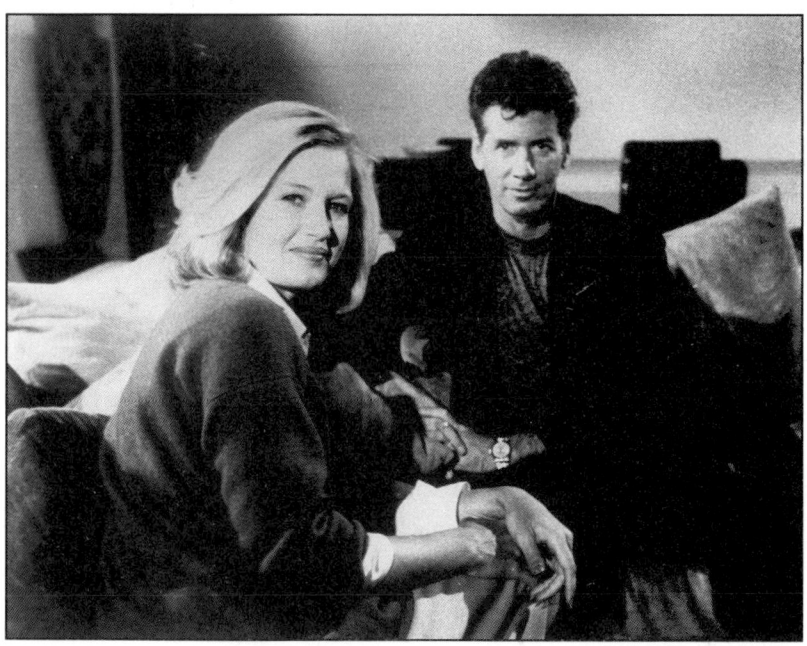

Diane Sawyer: Handsome Hair

less hierarchical, less careerist. Also, some believe the world of work in the '90s is different for women. They no longer have to demand their place (though pay and position are still at issue), and this means they may return to new and more sensual kinds of looks. They can give up the uniform.

On both counts, Brenda needs another haircut. Her '80s cut was too competitive, too formidable for the kinder, gentler '90s. Plus, her '80s cut was designed to demonstrate her competence in the world of corporate law, and that point is now clearly made. The time has come for something more expressive and less severe. Like the rest of us, Brenda is looking for a new self to match the new decade.

These five women in search of new haircuts deserve better than the stereotypes. In each case, we see them using their hair as the testing ground for new selves. Cynthia seeks a new personal style, Barbara a path away from her mother towards independence, Ruth a workable form of womanhood and Brenda a vision of professionalism. Janet would like to use her hair for self-discovery but her family is too threatened to let her do so. In our transformational culture, women use hair as the stuff of their metamorphosis.

"Mr. Antoine Will See You Now:"
The Old World of Hair

There was a time when hair was anything but transformational. In the 1950s, women wore their hair in beehives and bouffants, great towering hairdos frozen into place by permanents and hairspray. This hair gave no hint of fluid, mobile selves. This hair spoke of highly conventionalized, unchanging selves, of women frozen into place.

I glimpsed this first in a 1956 article from *Good Housekeeping* entitled "Spray to Make Your Hair Behave."[1] The article offered two photos as illustration. The first one shows a woman looking strange and stiff, a little like a mannequin. The second photo shows her wind-blown and lively, looking distinctly more dynamic and attractive.

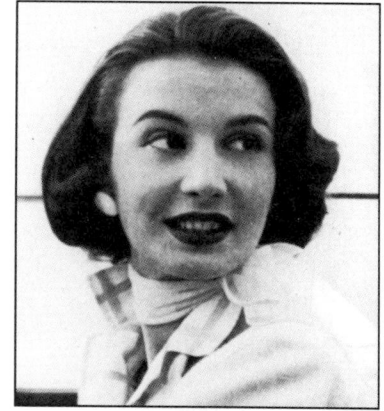
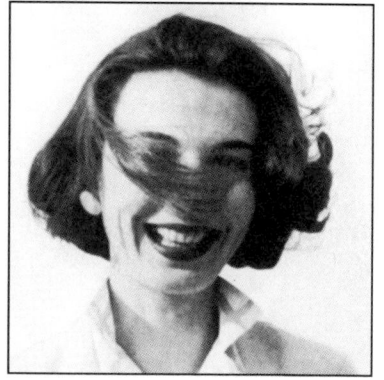

Spray to Make Your Hair Behave

Good Housekeeping hated the look in this second photo. They couldn't say enough bad things about it. They declared it "scrambled." They said it was a riot of "straggling wisps" and "flyaway strands…wrecked by the wind." To the 1950s eye, it had the very opposite of the "desired effect."

Women in the 1950s routinely locked their hair into place with hairspray, teasing and permanents. It didn't appear to matter that '50s hair was damaged, repellent to touch, that it made the wearer dependent on her hairdresser, that it demanded hairnets by day and rollers by night, that it was high maintenance all the time and never quite right. And it especially didn't appear to matter that this hair made women look terrible. It was as if they didn't have much say in the matter.

Sure, there was a place for women at Frank's

I fell to wondering about the old world of hair. If women's hair was a study in fixity, was men's hair more transformational? Perhaps transformation was somehow a gender privilege, something men insisted on keeping for themselves. Wrong again. If anything, the '50s world of men's hair was even more anti-transformational than that of women.

Take the barbers themselves. They were resolutely plain men, with names like "Frank" stitched emphatically above the pocket of blue, no-nonsense smocks. They all seemed to have the same look: no necks, a gruff manner and the world's shortest hair, like Phil on "Murphy Brown."

The barbershop was a plain place, too. Frank had three or four chairs, several mirrors, a sink, a calendar from a local hardware store, a dying plant or two, a coat rack, a radio and a drawer full of *Playboy* magazines. (Sure, there was a place for women at Frank's. As long as they were stripped of everything but a besotted look of sexual expectation, they were entirely welcome.)

Frank gave his barbershop all the charm and homeyness of a fishing cabin. It was systematically and deliberately deprived of taste. "Hey, we're only cutting hair here," Frank would say, if you asked him. "It's not a goddamn shrine to Athena." Pretense of any kind was unwelcome. "You want fancy-pants decoration, you want lah-de-dah manners, you go down the street. I think Mr. Anthony's got a three o'clock open for you."

As proof of his indifference to matters of style (and other instances of transformation), Frank specialized in the "short back and sides." And he was particularly happy when giving the crew cut ("that disease of the scalp," as Vidal Sassoon would later call it[2]). Typically, perhaps deliberately, Frank's cuts made his customers look like hell.

Conversation at the barbershop turned, often, on the fortunes and misfortunes of the local sports team. All of this was classic guy talk. Short sentences. Pithy observations. A carefully managed economy of thought and feeling. Men demonstrating they knew more than they were saying. No florid emotions, no dramatic declarations. Just short, sharp talk. Everything buttoned down.

But the radio did not always carry sports. If you were really lucky, Frank's radio would be tuned to the police band. What could be more male? Men talking to other

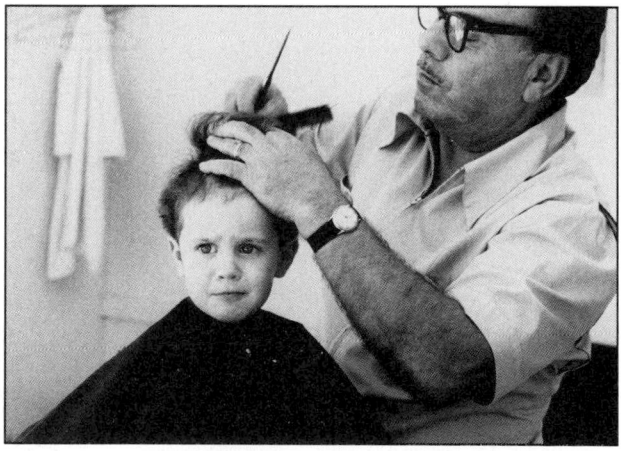

Anti-transformational hair?

men about emergencies that mobilized large groups of men in the execution of heroic action. The guys at Frank's listened with rapt appreciation and complete identification.

Conversation became positively telegraphic. Suddenly everyone at Frank's got pithy. "Sounds bad," "Could be the Johnson place" and, in a burst of free speech, "Boys, you got your work cut out on this one."

Hair in the 1950s, it turns out, was anti-transformational for both men and women. Both sexes treated hair as if it were a dangerous substance. Of course, they reacted differently: women with fastidious discipline, men with fastidious disregard. But both sexes showed an unmistakable nervousness in the presence of this

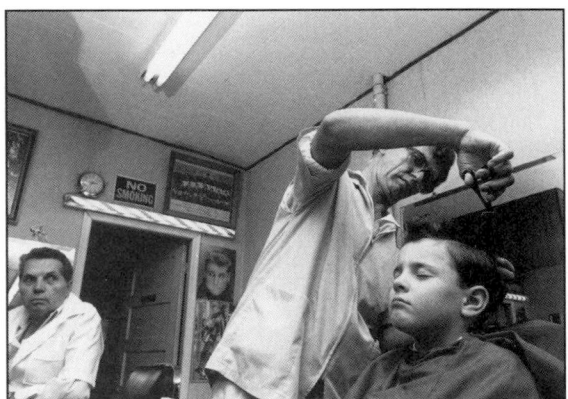

Induction into the cult of maleness

deeply disturbing thing called hair.

Getting to the bottom of this attitude is not easy. Why should hair have been such an alarming substance in the 1950s? You'd think they had enough to worry about in those days, what with the Cold War, sitting too near the TV, open-plan architecture, beatniks, bomb shelters, car ports, TV dinners, air-stream homes, Korea, Communists and keeping up with the Joneses. How could so natural a substance as hair have struck anyone as odd or problematical? It has to do, I think, with the constellation of values that defined the decade, and especially men and women.

In the war against nature, women were non-combatants

The 1950s was a decade that believed resolutely in progress, science, technology, rationality and experts.[3] This post-war period brought a flowering of new possibilities. Science and technology promised a happier tomorrow, new comforts and, most of all, the complete mastery of nature. The important frame of mind was the rational one. Art, intuition and emotion were not prized as ways of knowing. Scientific reason—that was the thing. As practised by the expert, this reason would buzzsaw its way through every mystery, every conundrum, every strangeness. It would help science serve its single, glorious purpose: to subdue nature and thereby extend the glorious technological dominion of man.

In the 1950s all of this was pretty much a *male* enterprise. All of this subduing, controlling, mastering—these were male enthusiasms. Science was a gender exercise as exclusive as football. Women could watch. Women could admire. But they could not play. In the war against nature, women were non-combatants.

Actually, it was more complicated than that, for it appears that women challenged, in a subtle and a not-so-subtle way, the entire male mission. They insisted on highly unscientific things like art, intuition, emotion. They claimed not to care about machines. They even claimed not to understand that local shrine of masculinity, the car. Their world tended, instead, to turn on things that were organic and sensual—on relationships, food, caring, children. It was as if women weren't really trying hard enough. It was as if they didn't care.

Intuitive, emotional and nonconforming, women were not just indifferent to the male enterprise of the 1950s, they were in some sense *opposed* to it.

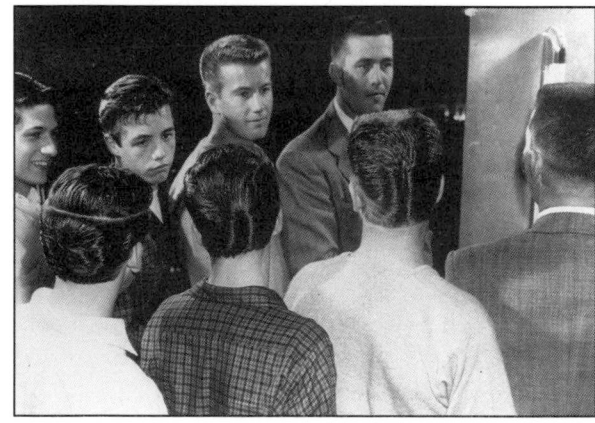

Men's hair in the 1950s

They were part of the unrepentant, the unobliging, the unco-operative natural world. And this made them what nature was: the enemy. If the 1950s was a time for science to seek the control of nature, it was also, willy-nilly, a time for men to seek the control of women.

Enter hair. Here was a perfect symbol of women (and nature). Uncontrolled, women's hair was everything women were: organic, expressive, emotional, spontaneous, transformational and sensual. Controlled, it was everything women (and nature) were supposed to become: meek, unthreatening, compliant and disciplined. Hair was the perfect playing field for the 1950s version of the war between the sexes.

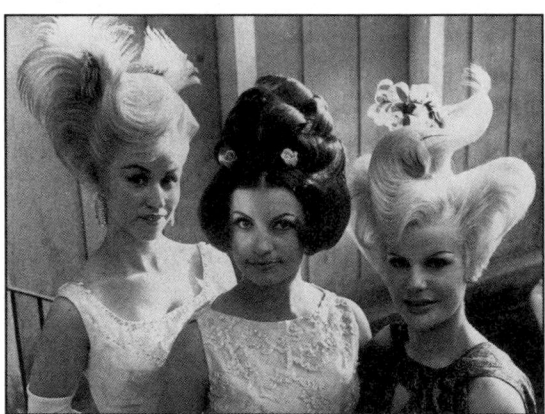

Women's hair in the 1950s

Enter *Good Housekeeping*. That second photo in "Spray to Make Your Hair Behave" was loathed by the magazine because it represented a woman who had escaped the constraints of the old world of hair. The most natural, organic, transformational part of her had somehow got free. The reaction was revulsion. This woman was AWOL.

Enter hairspray. When *Good Housekeeping* sung its praises, it was doing more than giving beauty advice. It was issuing gender instructions. It wasn't just hair that was supposed to "behave," to be "smooth, mannerly and disciplined" and to stay "meekly in place." Forty years of feminist theory later, it's pretty clear what *Good Housekeeping* was really saying: Spray to Make the Self Behave.

Enter all those '50s haircuts. Women were carrying symbols of servitude around on their heads. The bouffants, the teasing, the hairspray, the permanents—all of these were designed to lock hair into place. They were designed to imprison the sensuality, imagination and naturalness of women in a decade that wished to suppress them all.

And what to make of the barbershop? Why were men being so insistently masculine here? Why were they beating the drum of gender so loudly? In retrospect, it seems clear enough. They were taking precautions. In the presence of this strange, powerful, transformational and terribly female substance called hair, they were proceeding with care.

After all, they had made hair a symbol of things female. And now, to get their hair cut, they were having to *trespass* in a female domain. The barbershop was actually located on women's territory and men were doing what men always do in these circumstances. They were puffing themselves up. They were showing they were not afraid. At all. Not even a little. Really.

So they recruited guys like Frank, turned shops into a fisherman's shack, stuffed it with *Playboys*, brought in a police radio, talked about sports and policework with stunning economy and got haircuts that declared

A large, red, white and blue drilling phallus didn't seem to overdo it

an almost monk-like indifference to style. Could we be any more clear? We don't want anyone getting the wrong idea. We may be trespassing in the female world of hair but we are still males. We are still utterly untransformed, still resolutely men.

But a doubt still lingered. Was this place *really* male enough? After deep thought, men asked themselves, "Isn't there something more we could do?" And someone had a brain wave. What about a really vivid version of that medieval invention, the barber's pole? They made it red, white and blue, and they made it move in an upward, drilling motion. In the transformational, organic, powerful

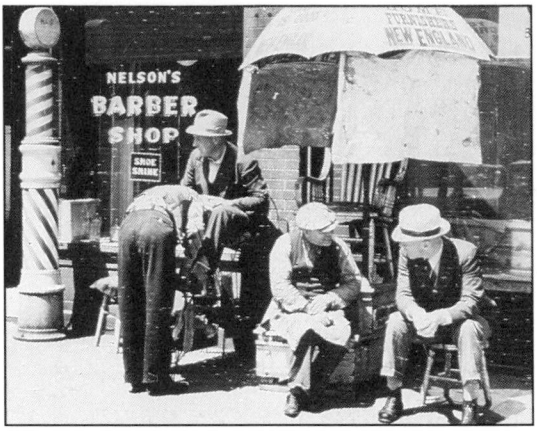

Reassurance of a drilling phallus

world of hair, where they were forced to leave off the comforts of science and rationality, men needed all the reassurance they could get. As far as the guys at Frank's were concerned, a large, red, white and blue drilling phallus didn't seem to overdo it.

The Princes of the Old World of Hair

Someone reckoned in 1958 that there were about a half million hairdressers in the old world of hair. It is a mark of how little the world thought of them that there is now almost no record of their lives. Only the aristocrats among them, all of them male, left a trace. These men give us a glimpse of the 1950s world of hair, and their stories illustrate a painful irony. These hairdressers were both agents of the anti-transformational male regime and the victims of it.

Ernest Adler

Adler was a young Jewish Bostonian who happened into the profession in the early 1940s and ended up taking it by storm. He invented a place for himself in the Broadway theatre world by force of personality, and eventually captured television, nightclub and Hollywood clients as well. In his time, Adler did the hair of Judy Garland, Dorothy Lamour, Patti Page and Betty Grable.

Adler was an unapologetic partisan of the practices that made '50s hair insufferable. He insisted on lacquering. He recommended a strict bedtime regime, involving clips, tissue, a hairnet and much wrapping and pinning, and of course the discomfort of a night in bondage. And he had no patience for those who refused the responsibility. "A woman has to work at it, every night," he scolded. Obviously, some women were sneaking off to bed with scant regard for the work of genius on their heads. For Adler, this was like using your Henry Moore as a doorstop.

However, even the most elaborate pinning and wrapping could not preserve Adler's creations. They were designed as great acts of artifice, and, not surprisingly, they wilted shortly after they left the master's presence. According to Maurice Zolotow, writing in the *Saturday Evening Post*, "The trouble with an elaborate Adler coiffure is that almost nobody but Adler can repeat it the next morning. Once slept in, it's gone forever."[4]

Adler liked to trumpet his abilities. He called himself an artist, "a sculptor of the head," as he liked to put it. From time to time he would also call himself a psychoanalyst. One visit to his salon, Adler claimed, was worth six trips to the shrink. Naturally, these two metaphors were wildly at odds. To claim to be both an artist *and* a doctor was to combine C. P. Snow's two solitudes of art and science at the very time when they were most mutually exclusive. But Adler didn't care. He wanted the world to know his working life was not a "trade." He wanted the world to know he was extraordinary.

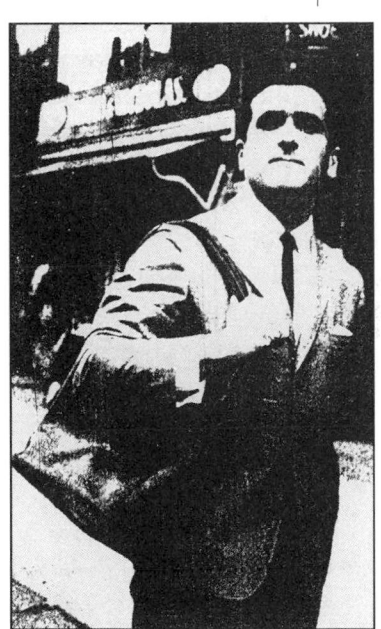

Adler: A sculptor of the head

Well, naturally, the male regime was having none of this. If hair was dangerous, hairdressers were worse. Here were men actually aiding and abetting women as they worked with this transformational thing called hair. At best, they would serve, as Adler did, to help women constrain the power of their hair. At worst, they were, potentially, traitors to their sex: men helping women escape the gender prison house created by their hair. Potentially, they would act as transformers.

Men worked swiftly to contain the threat. They declared male hairdressers ridiculous and *infra dig*. They forced them to surrender both gender and class credentials. Obviously, hairdressers were little better than gigolos. Or perhaps they were gay. In any case, declared the male regime, they weren't really "men." They weren't acceptable in polite society and they weren't acceptable at Frank's. Ironically, the men who helped run the oppressive old world of hair were, finally, rewarded by other men with character assassination and scorn.

These male hairdressers reacted as anyone would. They reached for anything that would give them standing. They claimed to be doctors. They claimed to be artists. But the strategy seemed only to make things worse. "An artist?" people scoffed. "A psychiatrist?" they mocked. "We don't think so." The cycle was inescapable. The more hairdressers were denied status, the more they sought it. And the more they sought it, the more it was denied them. They were trapped.

Journalists used rather less flattering metaphors of their own. Maurice Zolotow opened his 1958 *Saturday Evening Post* article by calling Adler a "swaggering little man" who looked, and acted, like "Napoleon." Here was another part of the cycle. As long as hairdressers were disdained, some of them would act as Adler did, by using gesture, tone of voice and facial expression to compensate for the world's low opinion.

Alexandre belonged to this new élite, the aristocracy of taste

They would seek grandeur in the small but crucial gestures of everyday life. This, too, failed. It was truly a no-win world.

Alexandre

Alexandre is another of the great hairdressers of the 1950s.[5] So great was his fame that he was known, like Sting, by his first name only. He too came from modest origins to make himself the hairdresser of the rich and famous. In Alexandre's case, this meant a crowd even more lofty than Adler's. Alexandre served European aristocracy and, most famously, the Duchess of Windsor.

But status remained a vexing issue. Alexandre used to say the Duchess "made me a gentleman," vaulting him from a French fishing village into polite society. But not even this

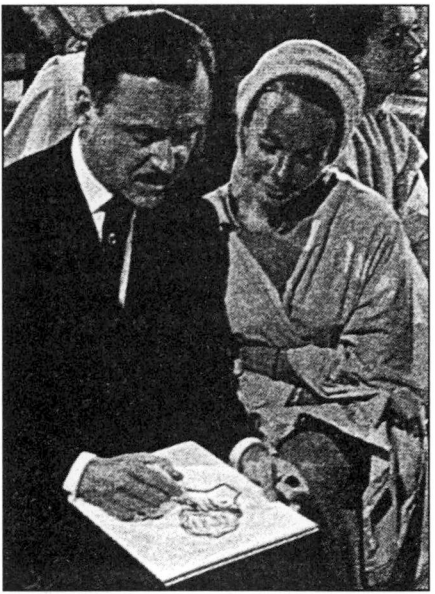

Alexandre: Just a hairdresser?

apotheosis could break him out of the status trap. He remained for all that "just a hairdresser." The lowliest bank manager could claim more status. The average schoolteacher could sneer. Both did.

Nevertheless, Alexandre *was* a man to be reckoned with. He did wield the most extraordinary transformational powers. Men might not have seen this, but his clients surely did. Even the most exalted of them needed him. Women of great beauty and prestige would refuse to appear in public without his ennobling attentions.

Sometime in the eighteenth century, the aristocracy had decided that they would make fashion a crucial symbol of their social standing, and from that moment onward, the likes of the Duchess of Windsor came to depend on the likes of Alexandre, a boy from a fishing village.[6] Alexandre belonged to this new élite, the aristocracy of taste, and on this score he ranked higher than even the most noble of his clients.

By the middle of the twentieth century, "birth" aristocrats had come to depend enormously on "taste" aristocrats. An issue of *Good Housekeeping* shows the changing hairstyles of Princess Margaret from 1948 to 1967.[7] These twelve pictures are clear evidence that the princess was always following fashion and never directing it. New fashions no longer flowed from the court. By the twentieth century, the old pattern was long past and the "gentleman coiffeur," as Alexandre liked to style himself, was in the ascendency.

This development made hairdressers like Alexandre a kind of parallel presence in the land. While the Duchess of Windsor was elevating Alexandre with her lessons in deportment, our hairdresser was returning the favour. By conferring new fashions upon her, he made her ready for polite society. He was endowing her with the aesthetic properties she could not live without. Without Alexandre's seal of fashion, the Duchess was, in the twentieth century

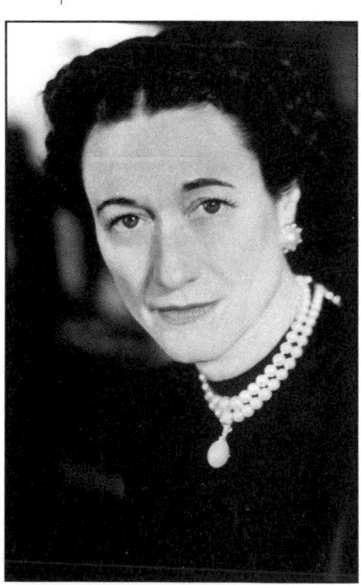

Duchess of Windsor: No aristocrat without Alexandre

scheme of things, merely a woman who had married well.

All of this gave rise to a paradox: a world in which hairdressers had precious little status but a surprising amount of power. In the Roman period it was not unusual for a woman to abuse her hairdresser, but by the 1960s, times had changed. *Vogue* captured it nicely:

Custom has swung round to a position which makes it unthinkable for a woman to say a harsh word to her hairdresser. Nor would she wish to; today's woman knows that she is only as chic as her coiffure—this is the acid test of fashion.[8]

By the twentieth century, the famous phrase "Without you, Your Majesty, I am ridiculous" belonged not in the mouth of Alexandre but to the Duchess of Windsor. A slip of Alexandre's scissors, a week of his neglect, and she was very nearly that.

The problem was plain enough. As a male living in the old world of hair, Alexandre would continue to be punished by other males. But as a master of the new transformational possibilities of hair, Alexandre would continue to be worshipped by his female clients. Alexandre was caught in a sexist society, between a male understanding of hair and a female one. He was subject to ridicule from the first group and gratitude from the second.

Antoine

Antoine was perhaps the most influential of the '50s hairdressers, but his career and his character bear surprising similarities to those of Adler and Alexandre.[9] Like the others in our triumvirate, he came from humble origins: in his case "peasant stock" in Russia and Lodz.

Like others before him, Antoine was irresistibly drawn to the dual metaphor of the artist and doctor. Ernest Hauser, his biographer, rewards him with patronizing punishment: "Curiously enough, when Antoine styles himself a creative artist, he is not really overstating things." It turns out that Antoine did some sculpting, and while Hauser is prepared to call his busts "credible" and "fair," the subtext fairly screams "Artist, right!" Once more the metaphor crashed and burned.

Hauser calls his article "He Domineers Beautiful Women" and marvels that otherwise sensible women could prostrate themselves before a man who was *only* a hairdresser. Hauser has Antoine's clients "obeying his wildest whims" and surrendering eagerly to his "sovereignty." Plainly,

Hauser could not believe his eyes. His article was haunted by the paradox that haunted the hairdresser: How does this man with so little status come to have so much power?

From a male point of view, the matter was genuinely mystifying. But it was utterly unmysterious to Antoine's clients. Plainly they truly loved, trusted and believed in him. Partly this was a reflection of his transformational potential in their lives, but there was another factor at work. Here was a man who was a kind of "honorary female." Antoine was sensual and expressive in a way most '50s males would not dare to be. Here was a man who had stolen across carefully watched gender boundaries to take up residence in one of the most important places in the world of women. And for his trouble, Antoine was punished as women were routinely punished. He was damned with the adjectives that men routinely used to punish and control women. He was declared flighty, dim, unskilled, unskillable and beneath any claim to seriousness. No wonder a bond existed. Antoine had forsaken gender privileges to join his clients in the ghetto. In the male regime, he and his clients were culturally twinned.

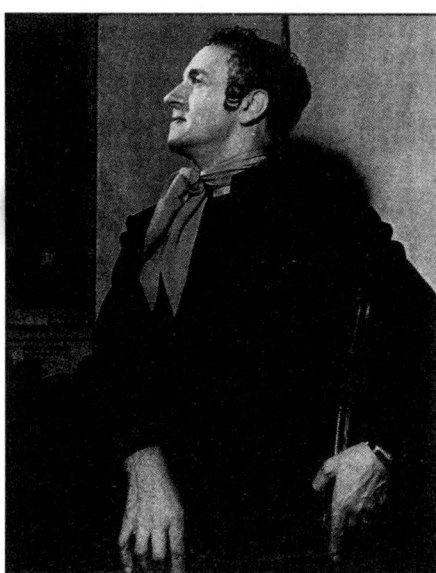

Antoine: Obeying his wildest whims

This old world of hair in the 1950s seems a long way away because it *is* a long way away. By the end of the decade, the end was nigh. A revolution was beginning on the other side of the Atlantic, and within a few years Vidal Sassoon would come ashore at Manhattan and take North America by storm.

Vidal Sassoon and the Great Leap Forward:
The New World of Hair

Vidal Sassoon opened his first salon in America in 1965. Strictly speaking, he needn't have. He was already influential beyond any hairdresser's wildest dreams. He was the famed originator of the five-point cut. He had created his own internationally recognized look. All London now acknowledged his genius.

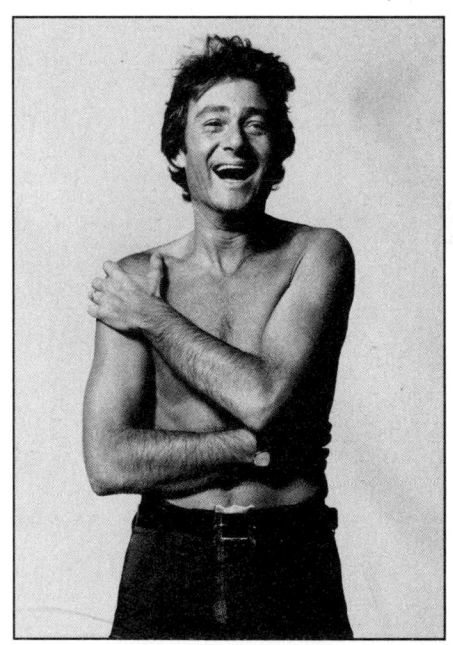

Vidal Sassoon

For some people this would have been enough. But not for Sassoon. He wanted more than local dominion. He wanted imperial power. He wanted to reform the whole of the old world of hair. This meant America.

It wasn't going to be easy. America was still very much in the clutches of big hair. Both hairdressers and clients were addicted to permanents, hairspray and teasing.

They continued, most of them, to believe devoutly in bee-hives and bouffants, fixity and artifice.

To his advantage, Sassoon could call on London's enormous cultural prestige as a fashion centre and the prestige of a career that had taken him from obscurity to stardom. He also had the backers, the ambition and the chutzpah necessary for the assault. But there was one thing he had not reckoned on: Judge Lomenzo, the bureaucrat in charge of the New York State Department of Cosmetology.

> *Before Sassoon could conquer the old world of hair, he was going to have to be certified by it*

No sooner had Sassoon established his Manhattan salon than the department summoned him. If Sassoon wanted to practise hairdressing in New York State, he would need the department's licence. And if he wanted the licence, he was going to have to take the department's exam. The irony was delicious. Before Sassoon could conquer the old world of hair, he was going to have to be certified by it.

Vidal Sassoon was not amused. He believed the Department of Cosmetology was an evil politburo. It encouraged hairdressers to practise the worst and most damaging ways of treating a woman's hair. In Sassoon's opinion, the department had made itself a gatekeeper, keeping in the bad and driving out the good. Sassoon left no doubt about his feelings about the Department and its exam: "The test requires that I do finger waving, reverse pin-curling and a haircut in which you thin as you cut — things that haven't been used since Gloria Swanson was in silent movies."[1]

Sassoon believed the Department of Cosmetology was committed to a wrong philosophy, that it encouraged hairdressers to think about a woman's head in exactly the wrong way. The department saw the head as a kind of platform on which the hairdresser built the "do." In this scheme, the client counted only as a plinth. In the cosmology of cosmetology, the client was merely the conveyor of the cut. She was merely the way a hairdo got into the world to win glory for the hairdresser. Sassoon was indignant. What about the client? No one seemed to care what she looked like or what kind of hair she had. Most important, no one cared who she was or where she was going.

And then there was the matter of style. The hairdos approved by the department were preposterous bits of rococo shrubbery that took their substance from permanents, their form from rollers and their rigidity from hairspray. They succeeded in making hair feel like a synthetic material. And for all their density and fixity, these hairdos proved to be enormously fragile and very

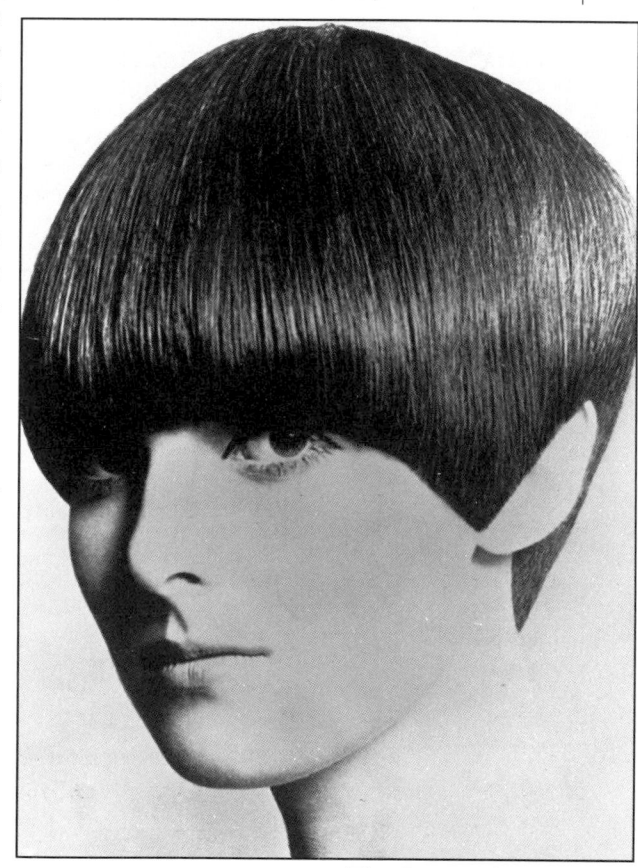

The famous five-point cut

high-maintenance. In the old world of hair, women were not just conveyors of the cut, they were also called upon to be its painstaking keeper.

The essence of the old world of hair was best demonstrated by the strange little lecture that closed every session at the salon. This should have been the moment when the client was asked how she felt about her new haircut. But instead what she got was admonishment. The lecture was always the same: Subordinate yourself to the do. This meant no sudden movements, no combing out, no crushing hats. It meant the endless strapping on of veils and scarfs. It meant sleeping with discomfort for fear of damaging the cathedral on her head. Who was wearing whom? In 1965 America it wasn't hard to tell.

Sassoon had a revolutionary view of things. You could see it in his own salon ritual. After a haircut, Sassoon asked the client to stand up and shake her head vigorously. Sassoon was looking to see whether the cut had captured the natural logic of the hair. Good cuts fell back into place; bad cuts didn't. He was also looking to see whether the new shape of the hair worked with the shape of the client. The idea that you could treat hair in this way was simply stunning. And what was more stunning still was the idea that you should care about the client in this way. The idea that the client mattered was, well, just plain astonishing. Plainly, an enormous change was in the works.

Ah, but the Department of Cosmetology and doughty Judge Lomenzo weren't having any of it. The department had its rules and its regulations. It had a public to protect. The department believed itself the last line of defence, the thin red line that stood between the public and the great untamed transformational wilderness of hair. Judge Lomenzo took the threat seriously. He girded his loins and pronounced from on high: "We're not going to be told what to do by these damn foreigners, especially these Limeys. Over there, you can't tell the difference between the boys and the girls!"[2]

We cannot know this for certain, but it's possible that the department felt a special antipathy for Vidal Sassoon. As an Englishman and a Jew, Sassoon was not once, but twice foreign. Even a modestly xenophobic administrator might see him as a threat. Sassoon must have looked like just the kind of guy who would disregard the rules and regulations (not to mention the gender distinctions) that the department was charged with upholding.

Double foreignness made Sassoon something more than threatening. It made him hard to discredit. If you attacked him as an effete Limey snob, Sassoon could present himself as part of the Jewish community that now controlled professional life in Manhattan. And if you called him pushy (that favourite code word of the xenophobe), Sassoon was also an Englishman who could damn you as a colonial hayseed. Sassoon proved a moving target and a frustrating one.

And this reveals what was probably the department's true motive in demanding that Sassoon take the exam. In the larger scheme of things, it would not have hurt to let one Englishman through the net. It had happened before; it could happen again. But this particular Englishman ... well, he was a little too galling. His philosophy poked fun at the old regime. His very haircuts cast doubt upon the depart-

The socks, if I'm not mistaken, are just a shade too short

ment's competence and legitimacy. No, Sassoon had challenged the department's authority too thoroughly to be absolved of it. The exam had become an act of deference from which he, of all people, could not be excused.

Just as inevitably, Sassoon refused the exam. It represented everything he hated in the old world of hair. So Sassoon said no. He would not acknowledge the department's right to control access to the world of hair. He would not acknowledge what he took to be their abuse of power. He would not acknowledge their bankrupt regime. He would make himself a conscientious objector.

In a 1966 *New York Times* interview, he declared, "I simply cannot take the test on the grounds that it violates everything I've worked for for 21 years."[3] Thus did Lomenzo and Sassoon come to engage one another in the old world of hair. It was a perfect standoff and a highly public one.

In retrospect, with the advantage of hindsight, it's hard for us to have any sympathy for the Lomenzo side of things. After all, there is something intrinsically odd (even unsettling) about using a bureaucrat to govern the world of style. Surely, the last person you want in charge here is a state official. In the last few years, we have learned to rethink government, to get it out of the places it shouldn't be (especially the bedroom and the marketplace). The idea that it ever presumed to control the world of fashion is too strange to bear contemplating.

Plainly, the Department of Cosmetology was never going to muster the subtlety or the aesthetic feeling it needed to be a truly useful or legitimate keeper of the world of hair. The evidence is everywhere. Where, for instance, do you think the department came up with the name "Cosmetology"? This sounds like something invented for the Soviet space program. Would it have been too much to ask for something winsome, lyrical or merely unridiculous?

And what do you think Judge Lomenzo was wearing the day he insisted that Sassoon write the exam? Civil servant shoes, possibly? Something in an indiscriminate Wallabee brown with those thick soles that look like ancient attic insulation? The ones with the "big weave" laces (look out, there's something on your shoe!)? The socks, if I'm not mistaken, are just a shade too short and the sans-a-belt pants just a shade too tight. He almost certainly wore the traditional upper-body badge of municipal office: wash-and-wear shirt, clip-on tie and jacket with lapels an inch out of date. And his haircut? I don't even want to think about it. Likely it was something turned out by Frank, the friendly barber. It might even have been a crew cut. And so he stands before us: Judge Lomenzo, lord of fashion, arbiter of hair. In the war to control the world of fashion, the Department of Cosmetology did not have a shred of plausibility.

Sassoon and Lomenzo had various supporters in their struggle. Predictably, the fashion press looked to be leaning in Sassoon's direction. Even before his arrival, fashion journalists had taken up the cause. Susanne Kirtland wrote an article for *Look* magazine in 1963 entitled "The Revolt Against Fancy Hairdos."[4] And Eleanor Harris wrote one in the same year called "Overteased Hair: the beginning of the end."[5] They had heard of the revolution taking place in England. They were ready for the end of big hair. They were ready for Sassoon.

Sassoon himself proved to be a master of the media. While Lomenzo toiled in well-deserved obscurity, Sassoon was busy claiming vast amounts of coverage in television, newspapers and magazines. At Roman Polanski's invitation, he agreed to cut Mia Farrow's hair in preparation for her part in the movie *Rosemary's Baby*. What made the event sensational was that Sassoon was paid five thousand dollars for the cut. America could not quite believe its ears. Five thousand dollars, for a haircut? The guy must be incredibly good. What made it even more sensational was that Sassoon cut Farrow's hair "live," as it were,

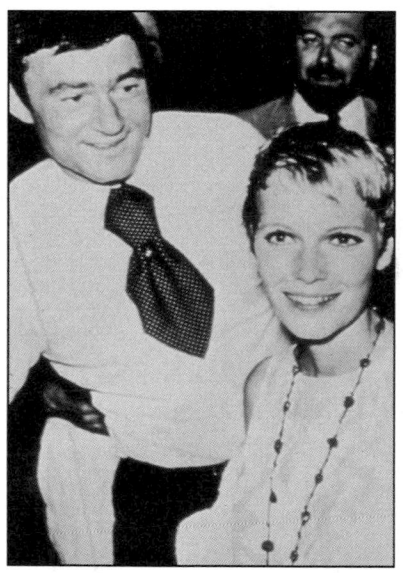

Mia Farrow's $5,000 haircut

on a sound stage at Paramount Studios surrounded by 150 representatives of the press, who shouted questions and jostled for position in what finally became a feeding frenzy. The world was mezmerized by the theatre of it all. Sassoon came away with a public relations bonanza.

Lomenzo might stamp his Wallabees in rage but there was nothing he could do.

But if Sassoon was the media's darling, the rest of America was largely on Lomenzo's side. The teenagers in Chicago, Detroit and Los Angeles, for instance, were utterly devoted to the "bouffant." Indeed, the style had grown to such proportions that some students could no longer enter school doorways with ease.[6]

In the old world, hair was frozen into place

Like these feverish teens in Chicago, most women remained in the thrall of the old world of hair, still very much the captives of big hair.

Sassoon's New Look

We know the outcome of this titanic battle. Sassoon won. The old world of hair collapsed. It came down like one of those office buildings that collapse in on themselves with one blast of carefully placed explosives. In the battle for share of heart and mind, Sassoon proved the more capable, the more cunning of the two. A revolution was underway. The new world of hair was born.

Sassoon proposed nothing less than an entirely new approach. He said to the industry, in effect, "Stop building hair out of artifice and additives. Let's build hair out of hair." Cut correctly, Sassoon showed, hair could serve as a foundation for itself, and you could dispense with the chemicals, rollers and hairspray. The message from Sassoon was simple but revolutionary: "Just cut it right."

Sassoon also demanded a clearer, more intelligent relationship between the head and the hair. He insisted that the hair ought to relate to the head, to correspond to its shape. This put the client back in the picture. No more "shut up, stand straight, and consider yourself lucky to carry this hairdo around on your head." Now the hairdresser was supposed to pay attention to the client.

Shaping the hair meant shaping the head. The hairdresser was now sculpting hair and client both.

The opening cuts were revolutionary. In 1963 Sassoon introduced the geometric cut. The bob, the V-shaped cut, the asymmetric cut and the five-point cut soon followed. I remember, in the early '60s, seeing my girlfriend in the five-point cut. I thought she was the strangest creature I had ever seen. Wisely, I kept this to myself. And I pretended not to notice when entire families would stop in the street and point at her as we passed. I grew to like the look. But it was the end of our relationship. She was suddenly worldly and sophisticated, and I was, just as suddenly, shambling and awkward and twelve. The Sassoon cut had transformed us both.

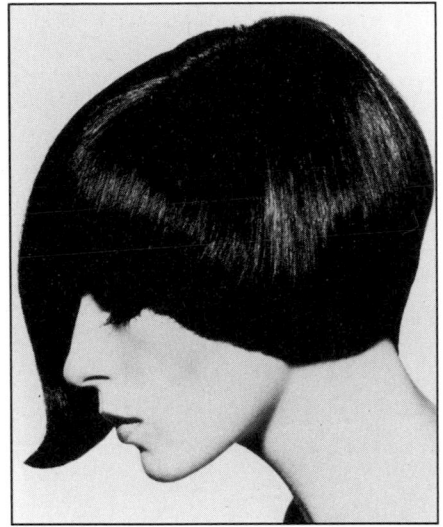

Asymmetrical haircut

One of the most telling comments on Sassoon's accomplishment comes from Mary Quant, his friend and inspiration. "He's a kind of Chanel of hair. He invented cut, swing, and fall. He was a total revolution." What a telling thing to say. These are, after all, natural properties of hair. To say that they had to be *invented* by Sassoon tells us how completely they had been

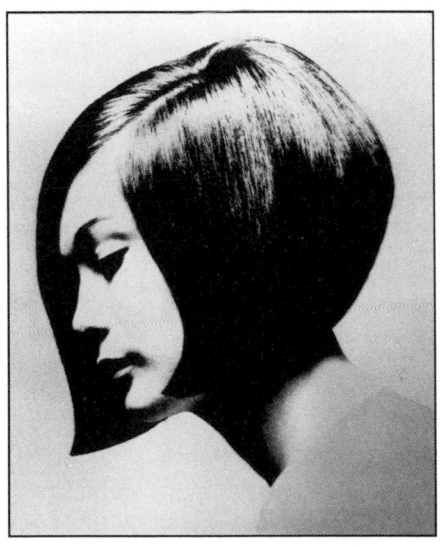

Nancy Kwan in an early Sassoon bob

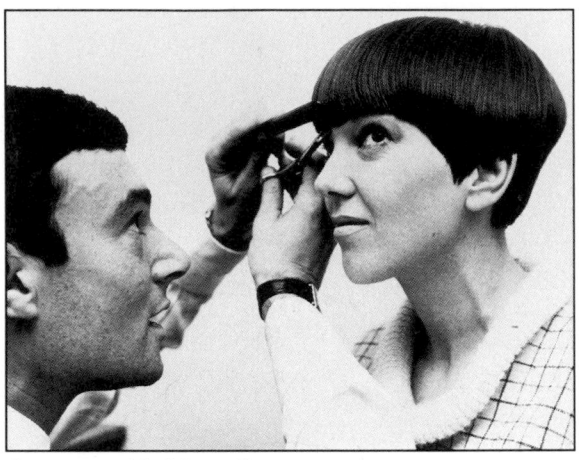

Sassoon with Mary Quant

locked away by the old world of hair. Quant's remark also tells us that Sassoon's revolution gave hair motion. In the old world, hair was frozen into place. Now it was meant to move as the wearer moved. It was to respond to the wearer, the environment and the moment. Hair could swing and fall.

Sassoon's revolution went well beyond hairdressing technique. It went directly to the spirit and the world-view of the 1960s. After all, this was a decade of *motion*. The '60s saw itself as a time for people to release themselves from social convention and constricting values. The decade made itself the champion of the individual, self-expression and freedom of choice. Hippies rose up to belittle middle-class rules and demand something more open and fluid. In the signature adjective of the time, the world was "swinging."

This word "swinging" had a strong sexual connotation. People began to ask one another (and themselves) whether they were "swingers" and "swinging." It was a question about sexual orientation, whether you engaged in group sex, and how slavishly you obeyed the laws of monogamy. It came down to a single question: Were you hopelessly square or did you swing? Were you trapped or could you *move*? The idea of mobility was beginning to shape every part of society. Swinging had become a prescription for change in virtually every aspect of contemporary life. Sexuality, music, clothing, decor, graphics, even politics all now moved.

Sassoon, to judge him by his own writing, is not a falsely modest man. He knows something of the world he has wrought. But he is also not a glory-hog, the kind of man who recreates history to serve himself. He tells us that it was not he but his teacher, Freddy French, who created the "swinging" look. In his autobiography, *Sorry I Kept You Waiting, Madam*, Sassoon says people used to mock French: "They did not realize that here was a man who was going to change hairdressing, sweep away the rigid, set look and replace it with something soft and simple, fresh, natural and swinging in every sense of the word."[7] Whatever its origins, Sassoon was the one who brought the look to prominence.

Some may balk at the idea that Sassoon was a maker of his time, but we would be wrong to think that he was merely its product. His transformation of hair in the '60s helped create that decade's transformation of mood and outlook. He invented hair that helped invent the age.

All in all, Sassoon got what he was after. He turned local influence into international dominion. He changed the face of hairdressing and, in the process, he helped to change the nature of contemporary culture. Some 30 years after his tangle with that angry little bureaucrat swathed in wash and wear, Sassoon's empire continues to grow. It includes 22 salons with some half a million clients. His four academies train over 15,000 students a year. None of these students is instructed in finger waving or the reverse pin curl.

Sassoon and Modernism

If you listen to the sages, Sassoon was merely an agent of modernism. He did no more than bring the modernist impulse to hairdressing, years after it had arrived in the world of built form, clothing and product design. Grace Coddington, a *Vogue* editor, is firm on this point. So are the contributors to a recent volume entitled *Vidal Sassoon und das Bauhaus*. And so are Richard Martin and Harold Koda in their introduction to the newly published *Vidal Sassoon: Fifty Years Ahead*.[8] According to these distinguished observers, Sassoon was a disciple of the Bauhaus movement, someone who sought to bring the "form follows function" principle to hair.

There was a time when Sassoon accepted this and declared himself a modernist. Who was he to argue with Grace Coddington and so flattering a suggestion? But more recently, he has taken a more careful and, I think, accurate position. In an essay entitled "My Way to the Bauhaus," he notes in his own work certain parallels to modernism without actually accepting the comparison. As he deftly puts it, "I like the exercise of attributing my original ideas of hairdressing to Bauhaus …."[9]

Sassoon's revolution *did* have modernist features, to be sure. He refused the distinction between form and decoration. And under his influence hairdressing finally broke with Antoine's antique notion of style as ornament. Sassoon integrated hair, head, style and wearer. To this extent, he is a modernist.

But observe the differences. Modernism was, after all, a grand ideological venture imposed from on high. It sprang from a vision of a new social order. It fought ornament because it emphasized social difference and celebrated hierarchy. The modernists wanted simplicity because it was democratic. Modernism was for *the people*.

But in point of fact, *the people* hated it. They refused the modernist motif in both clothing and cars. And they hated modernist buildings. They hated to look at them. They hated to live in them. They hated to work in them. Modernism turned out to be that socialist uncle who comes to visit, bringing with him grand philosophical principles but precious little consideration for the people on whom he has foisted himself. Modernism was a nice idea, but it was not a popular success.

Sassoon, on the other hand, *was* popular. His cuts did not come from any grand ideology, and they were not imposed from on high. His revolution really *was* for the sake of the people. Women embraced his cuts as a way out of the old world of hair. They wanted hair that respected who they were. Sassoon obliged them. Sassoon *can't* have been a modernist. He was too likeable, too accommodating and much too democratic.

We see an old reflex at work here. Golly, if we can claim Sassoon was a modernist we dignify his accomplishment. He is no longer merely cutting hair. He is now engaged in an aesthetic revolution created by intellectuals and world-famous architects. But the reflex is, as we have seen, a self-defeating one. The modernist comparison makes Sassoon a Johnny-come-lately to the modernist event. Worse, it makes him a mere imitator. Still worse, it conceals his true accomplishment: the introduction of new ideas to the world of hair and our transformational culture.

Why Sassoon?

Why was it Sassoon and not some other hairdresser who swept away the world of the coffee klatsch, the police radio and the Department of Cosmetology? The answers to this key question are well buried. There are no good records in the world of hair. The participants rarely kept archives. The accidents of memory have damaged what is remembered, while jealousy and politics have distorted the rest.

It might help to look at Sassoon's background. A commando for the state of Israel in the earliest days of its existence, Sassoon went to Israel in 1948 and saw active service in the Gaza Strip. It proved to be a formative experience. Sassoon was there to see Israel as it was being cobbled together out of a handful of ideas and all the peoples of the diaspora.

It helped free women from the nasty little prison that was the old world of hair

Next to hanging, there's nothing like military service to concentrate the mind. The first and most compelling question that occurs to people sitting in a foxhole, bullets flying overhead, is, "What am I doing here?" You need a convincing answer. In Sassoon's case, it meant believing that the chimera called Israel could become a reality, that this extraordinary historical experiment could succeed, that revolutions can happen.

It is also true that Sassoon was simply a very ambitious young man. His autobiography tells us that he was constantly seeking a signature haircut, a look that was recognizably revolutionary and identifiably his. This great compelling motive, the search for recognition, does not come from Sassoon's ethnicity, his nationality or his time. It is simply the engine of individualism, that impulse that western societies set free and then recapture, the better to transform themselves.

Why Sassoon? There is another reason. It has to do with being English. The English are quite prepared to make

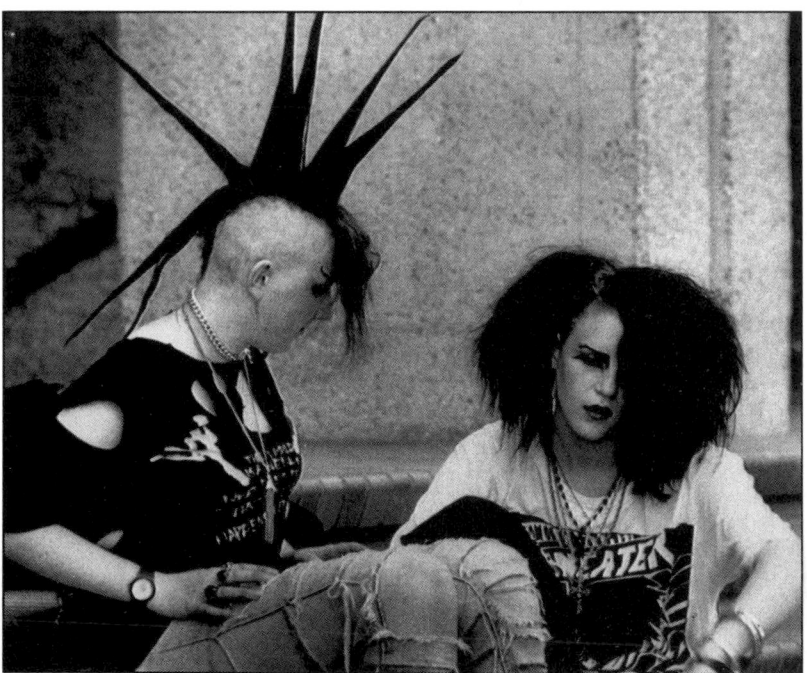

Fondness for the grotesque

themselves look grotesque in the name of fashion. This is not, in my experience, something the French or the Italians ever do. The French and the Italians will never let fashion disfigure themselves. Their fashion is never an act of self-defacement. But the English, some English anyway, don't seem to mind when the latest thing is not the most beautiful thing.

Punk is a good case in point. It made and still makes people look terrible. It deliberately violated conventions of prettiness, beauty, elegance. But punk is not the only example. Over and over, the English have embraced styles that make them look like hell. (I take Rockabilly, mod clothing and Vivienne Westwood's entire career as compelling evidence on my behalf.)

This fondness for the grotesque is a very useful thing for any nation that wishes to be a fashion originator. It expands the envelope of creative possibility. The "next thing" in fashion sometimes requires a violent break with the past. It is sometimes necessarily grotesque and difficult. Those who have a feeling for these qualities have an advantage. Sassoon has his own, characteristically less pompous, way of saying this: "In England, no one is scared to do something different. In fact, every English girl loves to look individual …."[10]

The glib thing to say is that Sassoon was the right man in the right place at the right time. But it's more accurate to say that this was a man with the endowments to create the time, place and opportunity. Sassoon began with a great act of self-invention and pressed on to reinvent the rest of us.

Sassoon's New World

Sassoon's struggle with the New York State Department of Cosmetology and the terrible Judge Lomenzo had many consequences. It helped free women from the nasty little prison that was the old world of hair. The iron hat of the bouffant was now gone. Hairspray and permanents, and the domestication they imposed, were now gone. Sassoon would be surprised, perhaps, to find himself called a feminist, but there can be no question that his revolution had feminist consequences.

Sassoon also changed the relationship between a woman and her haircut. In the 1990s, we simply accept that haircuts should help transform the self. This assumption owes something substantial to Sassoon's work. Before Sassoon, haircuts were, like many other things in a woman's life, an alienated, uncertain addition to the self. After Sassoon, they became, increasingly, the stuff of self.

Another consequence of Sassoon's revolution was a change in the status of the hairdresser. Sassoon's public persona in those early years was confident, exuberant, charming and tranquil. He was never seen to try too hard or to overcompensate. Sassoon was perhaps the first prince of the aristocracy of taste to behave like one. He did not storm around like Napoleon, he did not cultivate airs. He never called himself "Mr. Vidal." He never claimed to be a doctor or an artist. Sassoon saw himself as a master of contemporary fashion. He did not try to extort deference, and consequently it was given to him.

The most important thing that Sassoon's revolution accomplished was, perhaps, to break down the walls of gender segregation. By the end of the '60s it was all over. At the beginning of the decade, men and women had gone to separate salons. By the end of the decade, "unisex" was everywhere. Sassoon's revolution had tipped the landscape. Male clients suddenly poured into female salons, abandoning, as they did so, the old "fishing shack" barbershop.

The figures are catastrophic. Barbershops began to close. Between 1972 and 1990, they fell by almost half (from 110,000 to 60,000).[11] Men no longer looked to the barbershop and the stolid company of other males as the place to get their hair cut. Suddenly they began to enter the female domain of the salon. This was, to put it mildly, a very big change. And a very big irony. Isn't this just the thing Judge Lomenzo warned us about when he said "You can't tell the difference between the boys and the girls"?

Suddenly men were thinking about haircuts as a matter of fashion. They were beginning to see the advantages of style. Having long scorned women for their concern for hair, suddenly men were there too, sitting in the same chairs, looking in the same mirrors, listening to the same hairdressers. They had taken one giant step into the previously forbidden world of fashion. Sassoon's revolution was thoroughgoing.

But the single most important consequence of Sassoon's new world was that it made hair newly transformational. In the 1950s, hair was a strange and primitive substance to be feared as a symbol of wild and danger-ous femaleness. Now it was suddenly a substance that was *supposed* to change itself and the people who wore it. You no longer had to lock it down. You no longer had to ghettoize it. After Sassoon, hair became an official place of invention. It was becoming something that men and women would use routinely as an opportunity for metamorphosis. Hair provided the opportunity for an entire society to swing.

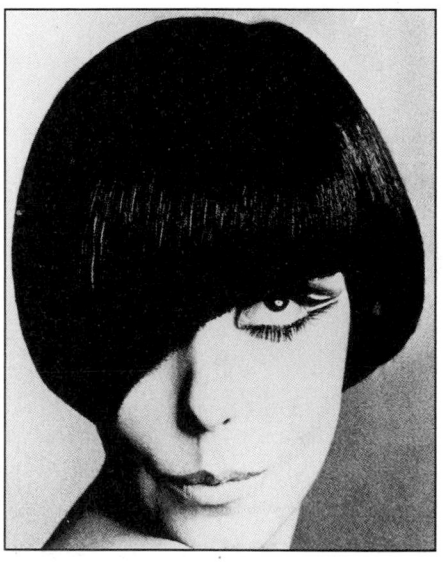

When Sassoon came to Manhattan in the early 1960s, he found himself in a familiar situation. Shades of 1948 — he was struggling to help establish yet another sovereign state. Resistance was ferocious. But it could not carry the day. Eventually, inevitably, Manhattan fell, and we all became citizens of a new world of hair.

Blondness: The Periodic Table

Monroe, Madonna and the
Invention of the Blonde

O nly one in twenty adult women are naturally blond. If it feels like there are rather more blondes around us, it's because in America four out of ten women add blondness to their hair. As a culture, we are obsessed with blondness. We have declared it the "essentially female colour."[1]

As a male, I feel the effect of blondness frequently. I'll be staring into space when somewhere, deep in my brain, a blonde-alert sounds. Suddenly, involuntarily, my head lifts, my eyes focus. I find myself looking

I hated the private school bullshit that pretends you don't have a body or a sex life

at a blonde. This is not because I am a blondness addict. It is not because I seek out blondness as some men do. It's because this culture has turned blondness into a beacon and wired it into the navigational equipment of every male.

But things may be changing. It's open season on blondes these days. They are the last undefended target in a politically correct world. "Dumb blonde" jokes circulate freely. The "blond bimbo" is mocked by both men and women. Once the colour of choice for American women, this look has new enemies.

It's impossible to tell how much damage has been done to blondness. If blondness were a stock, it would be too early to sell. We know blondness will continue as one of the most dramatic statements a woman can make with her hair, but we also know that the meanings of blondness are many and changing. What follows is a catalogue of some of the transformational possibilities contained in blondness.

Bombshell Blondness

"Bombshell" blondness is designed for the big effect. It is supposed to detonate in the viewer's gaze. It is designed to turn heads and stop traffic. Bernard's client Cynthia liked the look precisely because it was so attention-getting. She wanted you to know she was in the room. Bombshell worked for her like a fanfare. It gave early warning of the person to come. "You took one look at my hair, and you knew you were dealing with someone who had the volume turned up to eleven."

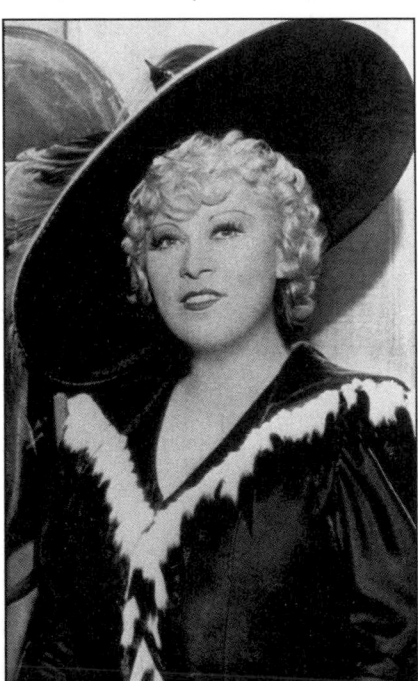

Mae West: an early inventor of blondness

Cynthia also liked the fact that bombshell blondness carries a sexual message. She is an openly sexual person, and she regards anything else as dishonesty. "Everyone is thinking sex a lot of the time. I hated the private school bullshit that pretends you don't have a body or a sex life."

The sexual message of bombshell was a long time in the making. It was invented by a series of Hollywood stars, including Mae West, Jean Harlow, Jayne Mansfield, Marilyn Monroe, Kim Novak and, more recently, Bo Derek, Brigitte Nielsen and Loni Anderson. And it is largely this sexualness that gives the colour its transformational effect, for better and for worse.

Bombshell blondness can still detonate. With its sexual explicitness, it can still turn heads and stop traffic. But it is also true that there is a rising tide of resentment. The "blonde" jokes are aimed especially at the bombshell blonde.

Repudiated by the feminists, the "dumb blonde" is the last acceptable target

> Q: How can you tell if a blonde has been using your computer?
> A: There's white-out on the screen.
>
> Q: How do you make a blonde smile on Monday?
> A: Tell her a joke on Friday.
>
> Q: Why do blondes have TGIF on their shoes?
> A: It means "Toes Go In First".[2]

The logic here is puritanical and sexist. It says anyone who is a fully sexual creature must be stupid. If you have given yourself over to the pleasures of the body, you must be immune to the pleasures of the mind. This is a traditional criticism of women as the "wild creatures" in our midst. We remain a culture with deep misgivings about sexuality and we are still prepared to punish anyone who is openly sexual. Repudiated by the feminists, the "dumb blonde" is the last acceptable target.

But it is also true that we hate the dumb blonde as one of the most insulting icons of a sexist age. This persona, we sense, panders to men's most exploitative expectations and their silliest insecurities. For some, the bimbo blonde bears an alarming resemblance to a blow-up doll.

Cynthia found this out the hard way. Her great dislike of bombshell is that it attracted the wrong kind of male— what she calls the "Yahoo element." There *are* men out there to whom bombshell blondness says "I am an object, treat me as such." And some people argue bombshell blondes are asking for this kind of treatment. They say that when the bombshell blonde invites sexual response, she must accept *every* sexual response. Surely this is sexist nonsense that absolves the male and blames the victim.

The blonde stigma is powerful enough to give some women pause. Here a woman reflects on the possibility of going blond:

> What stopped me was the fear that as a blonde I could misfire, and instead of being regarded as clever and classy, [I] would be dismissed as dumb and cheap.[3]

Notice that cheapness now joins the charge of dumbness. The notion is this: women who use blondness to make themselves look accessible make themselves too accessible. A suspicion surfaces. Perhaps this bombshell blonde is "easy," by which we mean she is accessible to virtually anyone. Now her moral character is also in question. The dumb blonde stigma has two thorns.

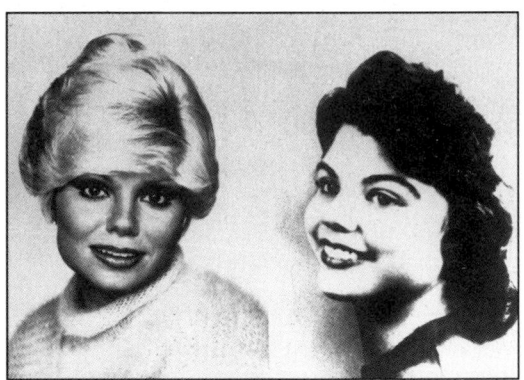

Loni Anderson: before and after the move to blondness

We have seen one or two attempts to reposition bombshell blondness in recent years. Loni Anderson tried in the television series "WKRP in Cincinnati." She played Jennifer, a receptionist with a helmet of bombshell blonde hair. By all appearances, she was the office "vixen." But Jennifer was in fact formidably capable, the only one at WKRP who knew what she was doing. The double message escaped some people. (Herb, her colleague at the radio station, never did quite master its "complexities.") But for others, Anderson helped to change what bombshell could be.

The bombshell image has changed so much that it is no longer, as it once was, a stairway to stardom. Hollywood is now littered with the careers of women who rose fast because of their bombshell sexuality and descended just as quickly. Joey Heatherington, Bo Derek and Brigitte Nielsen might be taken as examples.

The trick, apparently, is for the bombshell blonde to ride her sexual persona to stardom and then transform herself into something more lasting. Elke Sommer and Britt Ekland struggled to do this and failed. Suzanne Somers lived on past her television show "Three's Company" because she turned sexuality into personality. Claudia Schiffer, the Bardot-like

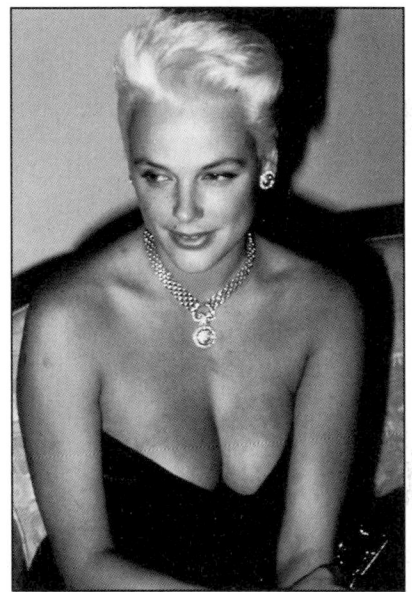

Brigitte Nielsen: Bombshell Blonde

model from Germany, is still an unknown commodity, but we do know that her kind of blondness, by itself, ages early. In our culture, you sustain this kind of blondness only by transforming it.

What is true for the star is true for everyone else. "Everyday" blondes are in the same predicament. They must supplement the first big impression with something more substantial and more interesting or pay the consequences. Once the detonation is over, only the stigma remains.

Sunny Blondness

"Sunny" blondness is almost the exact opposite of bomb-shell blondness. This look does not smoulder, pout or posture. There is no *vavoom* here. There is no overt sexual message. Sunny blondness is friendly, forthcoming and light. It is innocent, cheerful, open. It is, well, sunny.

Sunny blondes come bearing happy, open personalities, with just enough sexuality to steam the glasses of a fourteen-year-old male

Sunny blondness is designed to be *winning*. It sends a message of access, as all blondness does, but here access is not about sex, it's about emotion. It's about the blond opening up her thoughts and feelings. Sunny blondes are not supposed to harbour anything complex, manipulative, self-interested or dark. They are supposed to be simple, mild and innocent, in the manner of those great originators of sunny blondness, Doris Day and Debbie Reynolds.

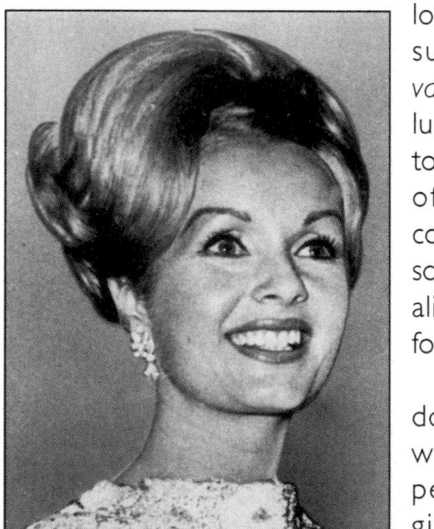

Debbie Reynolds: Sunny Blonde

Sunny blondes turn the sexual volume down quite low. It's there, to be sure, but sunny blondes do not do *vavoom* or anything smoky or lush. Sunny blondes are never torch singers. They are incapable of smoulder. Sunny blondes come bearing happy, open personalities, with just enough sexuality to steam the glasses of a fourteen-year-old male.

If sexuality is turned way down, "personality" is turned way up. Sunny blondes are perky and cheerful. We are given the impression that we know exactly what they're thinking: something cheerful, optimistic and friendly. The early Goldie Hawn, with her trademark "Laugh-In" giggle, was the perfect sunny blonde: charming, friendly, readable. There are, apparently, few mysteries to the sunny blonde. More exactly, sunny blondes create the impression that they are unmysterious when the truth is often otherwise.

We have seen a steady succession of sunny blondes: Cheryl Tiegs, Christie Brinkley,

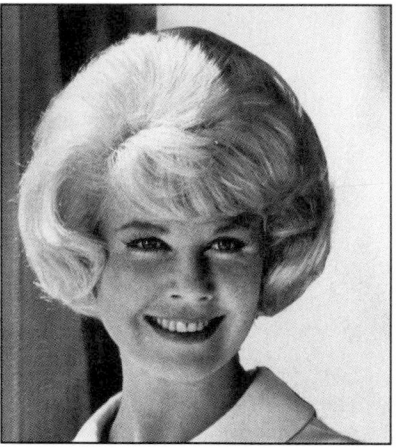

Doris Day: Another Sunny Blonde

Lindsay Wagner, Cheryl Ladd, Farrah Fawcett and Linda Evans. These women come to us from unmysterious sources like the hit TV series "Charlie's Angels" or the

world of modelling. Generally, they do not come from the more demanding worlds of theatre, sports or politics. All tend to play out the idea that women are simple and uncomplicated.

These blondes are never accused of being "cheap." Sunny blondes also last longer than the bombshell variety. After her scorching moment in the sun, the sunny blonde moves on to sponsorship duties for Sears or Revlon and gracefully enters middle age.

Lauren Hutton underwent this transformation. But as she grew more interesting, necessarily her persona grew less

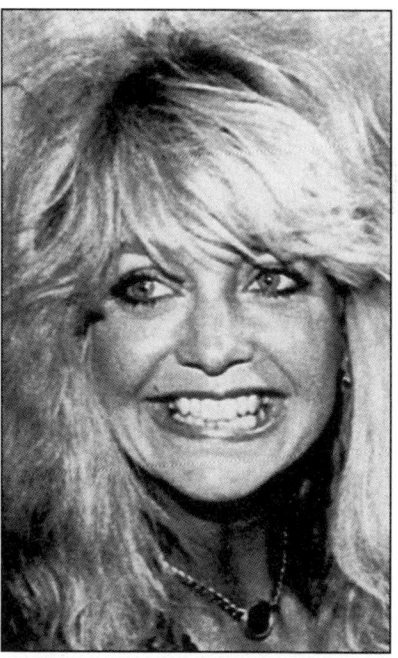

Goldie Hawn: A modern master of sunny blondness

sunny. It was a useful trade-off. Giving up sunniness allowed her to explore deeper, more complex aspects of her public self.

Women like Goldie Hawn have also rehabilitated themselves. Her persona is now miles beyond the happy airhead who contributed so much to the success of "Laugh-In." She is now an actress of ability. As a result, we no longer classify her as a sunny blonde. (Interestingly, we do not use Hawn as the occasion to rethink "sunniness.")

However, sunny blondness cannot be rehabilitated with ease. Many women do not want to appear more accessible and accommodating because this sunniness was for so long *exacted* from them. Sunniness may be a gender style whose time has passed. Unless it finds its saviour, this self and look will remain a minority look, and a diminishing one.

Brassy Blondness

"Brassy" blondes have big personalities. They are the ones you can always hear from the other side of the restaurant.

Brassy blondes do well as lounge singers

Brassy blondes do not mediate their feelings or modulate their voices. They switch on and stay on. If you don't see them coming, that's your problem. They had their hair lit up to give you fair warning, and if you didn't see it, well, next time, pay attention.

Brassy blondes do well as lounge singers. They are the kind of people who don't mind belting out show tunes in front of perfect strangers. They don't mind sitting in the lap of a nervous, balding man from Nebraska who hopes his wife is taking all of this in stride. Brassy blondes, according to the stereotype, are big-hearted, generous and kind. They have given away certain kinds of complexity and subtlety but they have done well in the bargain. They have purchased a candour and forthrightness that non-brassy blondes often wish they had.

Cybill Shepherd and Candice Bergen started as sunny blondes but we have watched them in the last couple of years move towards brassiness. The character Shepherd played on "Moonlighting" and Bergen's "Murphy Brown" have bright, big personalities. These photograph well on television, especially in the sitcom, where every emotion must be fully accounted for.

All in all, brassy blondness offers a nice compromise. It offers the "access" message that every variety of blondness does—you know exactly what they are thinking and where they stand—but there is no implicit offer of intimacy. The brassy self has a very clear boundary.

The current status of the brassy blonde is under review. This look was one of the ways women could make themselves heard in a sexist, male culture. This look gave you a certain power. But as sexism recedes, it is possible to have power and presence without forsaking subtlety and sophistication. Brunettes can wield the power of a brassy blonde these days, and they don't have to announce themselves ahead of time. Why give the game away?

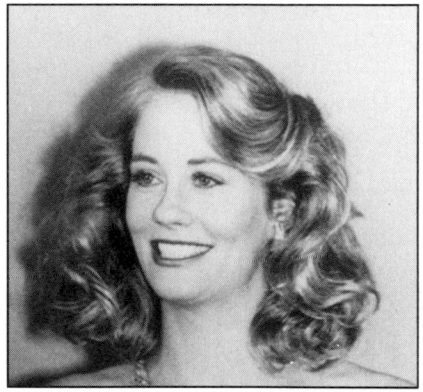

Cybill Shepherd: Brassy Blonde

Dangerous Blondness

One of the modern developments in blondness is the "dangerous" blonde. These are women whose hair colour offers access (sexual or emotional) and then snatches it away. I noticed this species of blonde the other day while I walked around downtown Toronto. For some reason, every blonde I passed seemed to be wearing sunglasses and a scowl. Scowling blondness struck me as an interesting variation on the theme.

A number of stars do dangerous blondness these days. Faye Dunaway, Morgan Fairchild and Sharon Stone are just a few. Dangerous blondes make good villains. Donna Mills on "Knots Landing" did it especially well.

Dangerous blondes are playing on the traditional symbolism: blondness as a statement of access. But the dangerous blonde seeks a statement of *qualified* access. She does not wish to be seen as "loose," and she certainly does not want to be considered "dumb." Nor does she want to be seen as transparent. The solution is *controlled* access, and that's what the dark glasses and the scowl are for. The blondness tells you "this is an accessible woman" and the dark glasses tell you "keep your distance until I give you permission to approach."

Sharon Stone built an entire career by being a dangerous blonde

There is a contradiction in dangerous blondness, but it's an intentional one. Women want to send the blondness message but they do not want to be penalized for it. When Donna Mills wears dark glasses, she is sending carefully contradictory messages. She is saying, "I am open, guileless and trustworthy," while she offers us the veiled gaze of calculation.

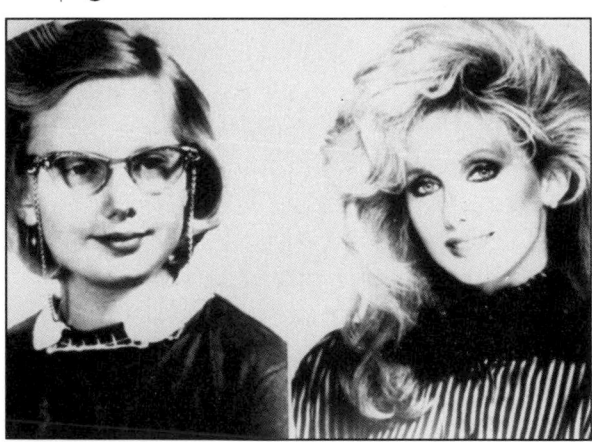

Morgan Fairchild: From innocence to Dangerous Blonde

Sharon Stone built an entire career by being a dangerous blonde. Famous roles in the films *Total Recall* and *Basic Instinct* show her as devious, manipulative and unscrupulous. One of the reasons that Stone plays these roles so well (besides her maturing talent) is that she is playing off her blond hair. We expect blondes to be agreeable, charming, accessible. Stone surprises, scandalizes and titillates us by being the opposite.

In this sense, dangerous blondes have cast themselves against type. It makes for a shocking effect. Some men find this intriguing—a challenge and an invitation. And audiences love the contradiction. Innocence and danger in a single package!

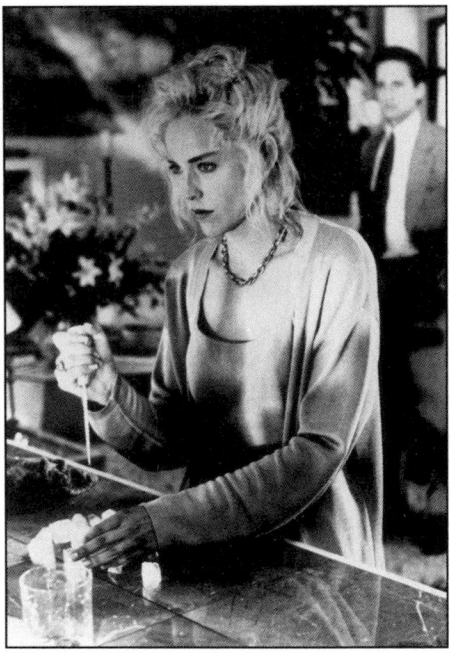

Sharon Stone: Dangerous Blonde

Society Blondes: The Platinum Blonde

When blondness goes "platinum" it takes on status meanings. According to Paul Rudnick, platinum was, for a while, the colour of choice for society women in New York City.[4] It was, and for some it remains, the look of choice on Manhattan's Upper East Side, Atlanta's Buckhead, Detroit's Grosse Point, Toronto's Rosedale, Vancouver's Shaughnessey. Platinum blondness graces some of the most elegant, best-coiffed heads in North America.

Platinum blondness has come a long way. Vilified with the terms "bottle blond" and "cheap blond," this colour has spent time on the wrong side of the tracks. It was close enough to bombshell to be a declaration of loose morals and a flag of promiscuity. To make it all the way to the Upper East Side took some doing. This is the Cinderella story of blondness.

Rudnick suggests that society women become blond to fight advancing age. Blondness, he says, softens the features. But there is another explanation. Platinum is a way for a woman to show the transformations of wealth and status.

Platinum blondes are telling us that they have graduated in the world. They are no longer beautiful young things. Having entered late middle age, they have cultivated other qualities. They have grown in wisdom and character. More particularly, they have grown in presence, grace and dignity.

What is the colour of dignity? It is most certainly not bombshell blondness—the sexual volume is up too high. And it cannot be sunny blondness—this colour is too eager. It certainly cannot be red, which is too exuberant and irreverent, or black, which is too cruel a contrast with ageing skin. And it can't be brown hair, which is said to lack presence.

There's only one choice: platinum. This colour skilfully harnesses the best parts of blondness and jettisons the rest. It engages light. It demands attention. But it does so with subtlety and a proper air of indifference as to whether the attention is

New York society never forgave Ivana Trump

forthcoming. Platinum blondness may tone down the sexual and emotional message, but it has found a new, more important one to put in its place.

Platinum blondness goes a step further. It claims a new kind and scale of value—deeper, more subtle qualities. It's as though the blonde is, like any beautiful object, taking on a patina.[5] Bright, obvious, look-at-me blondness has been extinguished. A darker, richer shade emerges and speaks of the new maturity, presence and dignity within. Blondness has been mined, the dross removed and the best grade of blondness made manifest.

But platinum blondness is only sometimes the real thing. It is often counterfeit, worn by women who have not completed a transition in grace and character. Some platinum blondes are "in training," as it were, and some are "bottle blondes" in the most disreputable sense of the term. Unwilling or unable to make the transition to new presence and grace, they seek to trick us.

New York society never forgave Ivana Trump, for being, well, Ivana Trump. They called her "Ivana Tramp," ridiculed her extravagant style of dressing and mocked her extravagant interiors. What they especially disliked was that Ms. Trump refused, for her own good reasons, to move from bombshell to platinum and to grace.

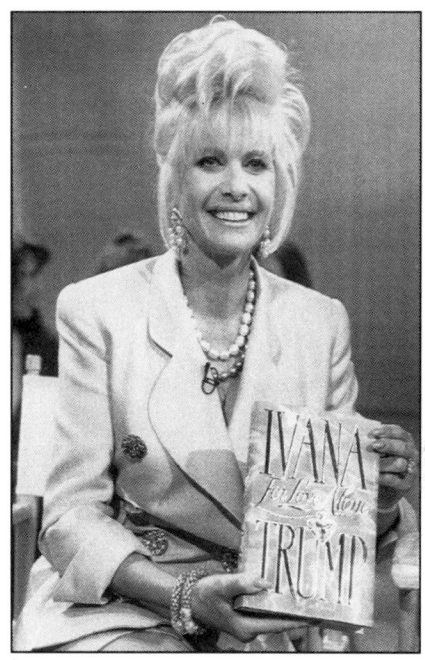

Ivana Trump: Fugitive from platinum

The Cool Blonde

One group of blondes has succeeded in turning blondness inside out. Consider Diane Sawyer, for whom blondness is a statement of distance and detachment. These are blondes who turn down the volume of emotional and sexual access completely. Indeed, they use their blondness as a statement of the opposite qualities. Sawyer's blondness is about reserve. Meryl Streep also does a very good "cool" blonde.

Cool blondes are a kind of puzzle. They are a little like dangerous blondes: they appear to be turning their backs on the very message of access for which blondness is so famous. And we find ourselves caught in the same contradiction. Our first reaction is to the "access" message of the blondness, and then we discover that this message has been turned right down. Refused, in fact. Cool blondness says, "Make no silly assumptions about access with me, kiddo."

This is not to say that cool blondes are not sexual. On the contrary, they manage an unmistakable sexual message. But you have to find it out. This has a charm all its own. It takes more subtlety to send this message and more subtlety to receive it. It is, as a result, a good way to edit certain males out of one's life. The cool blonde sends her message only to those with intelligence enough to hear it.

Hitchcock's blondes are so cool, so positively Nordic, they appear actually to have renounced their sexuality

The cool blonde was constructed, in part anyway, by Marlene Dietrich. Dietrich played her sensuality and her sexuality with great detachment. In *The Blue Angel* (1930), the film that brought her to stardom, Dietrich plays the blonde as morally lax gold digger. She bewitches a university professor, then, in short order, beds, marries, humiliates and discards him. The professor dies of a broken heart. Moral: beware the predatory blonde who would feed upon the naïvety of a good-hearted man.

Marlene Dietrich gave us blondness with eyebrows well arched. She wanted you to hear her sexuality but to know that she was not its captive. She wanted you to know that she could turn the turbines of sexuality on and off as she wanted. Marilyn Monroe made a happy, thoroughly innocent gift of her sexuality. Dietrich was somewhat more measured and calculated about the

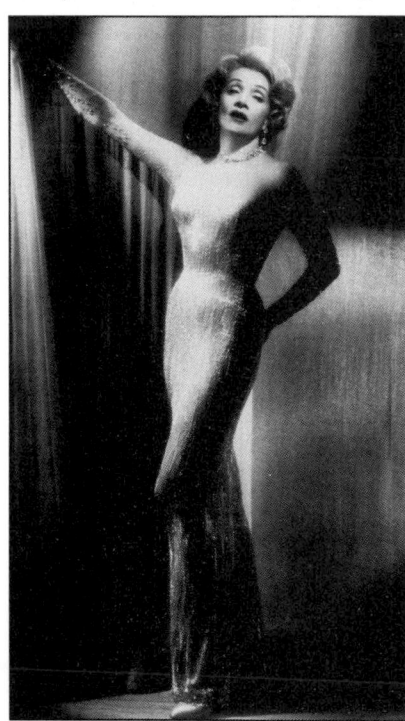

Marlene Dietrich: Cool Blonde

whole thing. There was no real generosity and no real abandon. Dietrich kept her distance.

The other person who helped to construct the cool blonde was Alfred Hitchcock. Sir Alfred is famous for a series of blondes: Madeleine Carroll (*Thirty-Nine Steps*), Grace Kelly (*Rear Window*), Tippi Hedren (*Marnie*), Kim Novak (*Vertigo*) and Ingrid Bergman (*Spellbound*). Hitchcock's blondes are so cool, so positively Nordic, they appear actually to have renounced their sexuality. These characters are as far as you can get from Mae West and the bump-and-grind extreme of blondness.

It wasn't that Hitchcock had no sexual feeling for these women. More than one of Sir Alfred's heroines complained that her relationship with the director was complicated by sexual tension. And it wasn't that he wanted them to forswear their sexuality on the screen. What he wanted was a

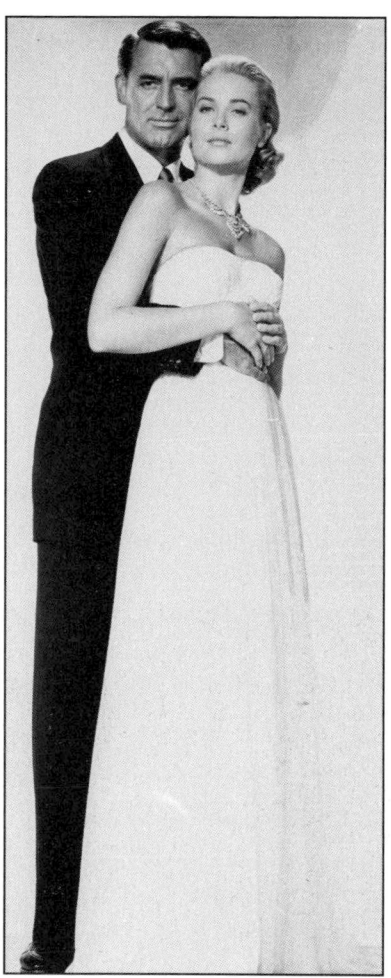

Grace Kelly: Cool Blonde in To Catch a Thief

tension between the sexual and the social. He wanted everyday life to be haunted by a sexuality that became all the more powerful for its annexation. Hitchcock began with blondness, the better to communicate a sexual presence, and then he directed the blondes to stand away from their sensuality. He sought to heighten sexuality by distancing it. (I'm told this makes more sense if you're English.)

Monroe: Mother of All Blondness

These many versions of blondness come mostly from the efforts of Marilyn Monroe, perhaps the most important architect of blondness in our culture. But Monroe invented more than blondness. She also invented a self to go along with it. As it turned out, she could not do one without the other.

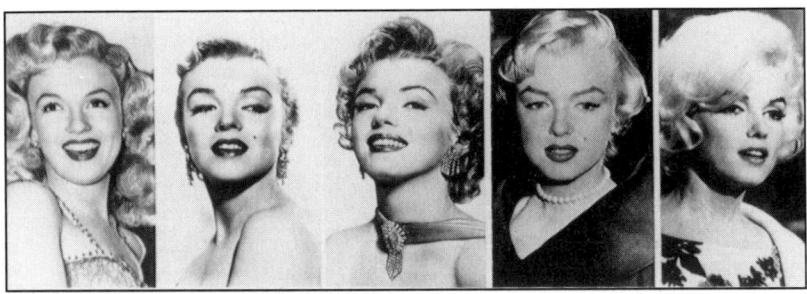

Marilyn Monroe was a classic self-inventor; she devoted much of her life to cultivating the creature called "Marilyn." But "Marilyn" was only a part-time self. Eli Wallach watched in astonishment one day as Monroe, on the street, suddenly began to walk and talk with new emphasis. The effect was electric. Heads turned, traffic stopped. Wallach asked her what she was doing and she replied, "I just felt like being Marilyn for a moment."[6] "Marilyn" was a special creation, not the essential self. "Marilyn" was an aggregate of symbols and meanings that suddenly took life and walked from the laboratory of Hollywood into our culture and our lives.

Making "Marilyn:" All the Cooks in the Kitchen

Monroe was not the only one trying to create "Marilyn." The press, the public, husbands and Hollywood producers all wanted a hand.

The Hollywood moguls, for instance, wanted to play the star-maker. The public had its own idea of who "Marilyn" was. (Manifestly, she was "one of them," a little person who had made it big.) Husbands had demands to make: Joe DiMaggio wanted his Monroe wifely and demure; Arthur Miller wrote her dumb blonde parts.[7] The press was (and remains) a relentless inventor of "Marilyn."

Monroe was not the only "Marilyn"-maker, but she was probably the most sophisticated and cunning of them. This surprises us a little. Monroe gave us the dumb blonde routine and we fell for it. It's hard for us to believe a "bimbo" invented one of the most arresting identities of our century. But as the biographies make plain, this was a woman who knew what she was doing and went about the business of self-invention with determination and skill.[8]

How Monroe Made "Marilyn"

If Marilyn was an invention, then the question is "How did she do it?" The answer is surprising: with every single resource at her disposal.

She began by changing her name from Norma Jean Baker to Marilyn Monroe. She got a new nose and chin. She gave up gingham sundresses. She changed her voice, facial expressions and body movements. Monroe even reinvented her history, claiming to have been a "little orphan girl" when this did not quite tell the entire story. And she changed her hair, from curly brunette to wavy blond.

All this careful invention got her somewhere. People raved. Leon Shamroy, the cameraman who shot her first screen test, said, "I got a cold chill. This girl had something I hadn't seen since the days of the silent pictures; this girl had sex on a piece of film like Harlow had. Every frame of that film radiated sex ..."[9]

"Marilyn" was a creature of Monroe's own making

There's a great temptation to suppose that this sexual charisma was somehow a force and a gift of nature; that Monroe was a passive vessel for something beyond her control. Even Steinem (who does more than anyone to let us see Monroe as a real person) stumbles on this point.

She speaks of Monroe's "extraordinary luminescence," as if this quality were somehow an accident of birth. And Norman Mailer, who can be relied upon to mythologize, talks as if Monroe were the completely witless recipient of extraordinary sexual powers.

This is nonsense. Worse than that, it is patronizing nonsense. The same biographies are filled with evidence that "Marilyn" was no gift of nature but the deliberate, thoughtful creation of Monroe herself.

One of her photographers saw this clearly. He could tell that even her white-light sexuality was no simple gift but a deliberate creation:

> I'll focus on her and then looking in the finder, I can actually see the sex blossoming out, like it was a flower. If I'm in a hurry and want to shoot too quickly, she'll say, "Earl, you shot it too quick. It won't be right. Let's do it again." You see, it takes time for her to create this sex thing.[10]

There is plenty of other evidence that Monroe worked hard to cultivate her persona. We are told that Monroe routinely took photographs home at night and examined them for hours. A young girl's vanity? More probably it was a young actress's craft. Monroe returned each morning to ask why some shots worked and others didn't.

Monroe tells us she sought charisma by deliberate craft:

> My God, how I wanted to learn! To change, to improve! ... I sneaked scripts off the set and sat alone in my room reading them out loud in front of the mirror. And an odd thing happened to me. I fell in love with myself—not how I was but how I was going to be.[11]

Monroe wasn't born with sexual charisma nor did she have it thrust upon her by Hollywood. Husbands, producers and the public all wanted a hand, but "Marilyn" was a creature of Monroe's own making.

Blondness Before Marilyn

To invent herself, Monroe needed to reinvent blondness. In the late '40s, blondness was not yet *the* colour of Hollywood. The movie stars of the period were mostly brunettes or redheads. In the silent movies, blondes were the exception, not the rule. The two greatest stars of the period, Lillian Gish and Clara Bow, were no blondes. Jane Russell, the reigning star of the pre-Monroe period, was a brunette. So was Katharine Hepburn. Joan Bennett began her career as a blonde but rose to stardom as a brunette. Rita Hayworth and Maureen O'Hara were both redheads. True, there were a few blondes with influence: Veronica Lake, Mary Astor and Joan Crawford, for instance.[12] But blondness was not then, as it became in the '50s and '60s, the starlet's choice.

There was, in fact, something slightly outré about blondness in the '30s and '40s. It was, after all, associated with Jean Harlow and Mae West. It was associated with frank sexuality in an era when any kind of sexuality made people a little nervous.

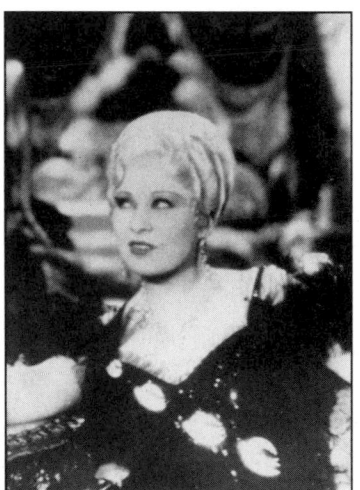

Mae West bears some of the responsibility. She helped to make blondness stand for sex on the sly. Her character came straight out of vaudeville, designed to radiate the stripper's coyness. Mae West's vamp helped to make blondness stand for sex as a naughty secret.[13]

Jean Harlow was not so different. She was, in Molly Haskell's words, "one of the screen's

Mae West with a leer

raunchiest inventions ... sluttish and smart, cracking gum and one-liners simultaneously."[14] She too helped to make blondness stand for a provocative brand of sexuality. Under the influence of West and Harlow, blondness became a declaration of wantonness.

Monroe's self-invention called for something different. At first, she didn't want to become a blonde at all. She had to be persuaded by her agent, the improbably named Emmeline Snively. Monroe was afraid blondness would look "artificial" and vampish, and this was not what Monroe wanted for "Marilyn." Mae West and Jean Harlow had charged it with a sexuality she did not want and could not use.

Marilyn Monroe was looking for a different version of sexuality. And because it was not available, she had to create it. She set about doing so in the movie *Gentlemen Prefer Blondes*. By the time the film entered popular consciousness, no one would think of sexuality or blondness the same way again.

There's an irony here. After all, the title *Gentlemen Prefer Blondes* was meant to strike you as odd and paradoxical. Gentlemen, everyone knew, preferred brunettes. Blondes were for the dance hall, the burlesque house. Blondes, in the tradition of Harlow and West, were creatures that "gentlemen" did not date, marry or, strictly speaking, even talk to.

Monroe managed her triumph right under the nose of the preeminent star of the period, Jane Russell. Russell came to the picture as the acknowledged star. She got bigger billing and more money (more than five times

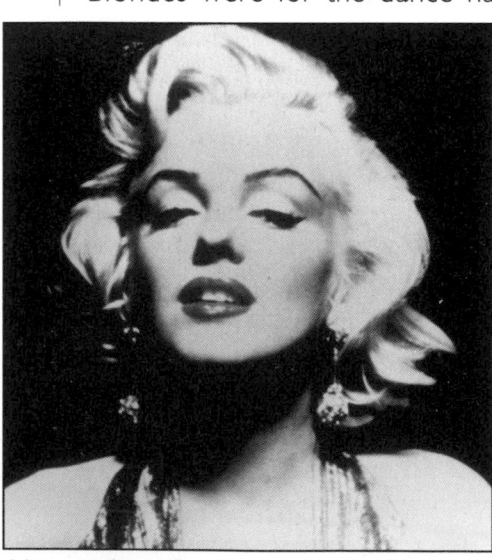

Monroe from Gentlemen Prefer Blondes

Monroe's fee). But the movie slipped away from her. She had the satisfaction, towards the end of the film, of donning a blond wig and doing a crude satire of Monroe's breathy innocence. But this must have been a fleeting pleasure. The picture belonged to Monroe.

A blonde rises, a brunette is eclipsed. By the time Monroe was finished, *Gentlemen Prefer Blondes* no longer had an ironic ring. It's true, the nation said, gentlemen *do* prefer blondes. Doesn't everybody?

The Myth of the Dumb Blonde

People have called Monroe's part in *Gentlemen Prefer Blondes* a "dumb blonde" role.[15] What they are complaining about are the mannerisms of Monroe's Lorelei Lee. She is breathy, pouting, wide-eyed, prone to grammatical error, constantly surprised by the world and unsophisticated in everything she does. These are, no doubt, markers of stupidity in some people. They are also markers of submission in a sexist society and, these days, we cringe to see them in the character of any woman, on screen or off.

But Monroe intended them for another purpose. What she was doing in *Gentlemen Prefer Blondes* was establishing a form of femaleness that was utterly unguarded. Her Lee is open and unmediated. This is the famous "vulnerability" that everyone always remarks on. Despite the fact that this creature is hot on the "millionaire trail," she is with everyone, from captains to waiters, a creature without boundary. Everyone has access to her emotions. She keeps no inner counsel. She cultivates no managed interior.

What the critics take for dumbness is, I think, the carefully cultivated access. And this was the quality that Monroe most sought for her invented self. "Marilyn" was charming because there was nothing measured about her, nothing calculated, nothing manipulated. Even the pretentions were transparent.

What was extraordinary about "Marilyn" was that she gave so much and demanded so little. All the rules of reciprocity were violated. The viewer was given access to the entire person. This was a person you could see right into and possess completely.

Naturally, we are, in an era reconfigured by feminist understanding, uncomfortable with this. We see now how dangerous the posture is, especially when it is practised by women, and most especially when it is demanded of women. From a feminist perspective, it is impossible not to see Monroe's "generosity" as something coerced. In Monroe's time, and in our own, the gesture is a dangerous one, a "gift" extorted from the giver and therefore not a gift at all. "Marilyn" was, and remains, an invitation to exploitation.

Liabilities aside, this persona was not like anything America had seen before. "Marilyn" was about access of every kind: sexual, emotional, intellectual. And America was smitten. The people were drawn to this selfless creature like moths to the flame. They came driven by many different motives, some exploitative and sexist, some not. America responded to the free gift of access as they do to any perfect gesture of generosity—with a generosity of their own. They gifted Monroe with stardom.

But Monroe also cultivated a new notion of sexuality. The sexuality of Lorelei Lee is an innocent sexuality. This was a frankly, openly sexual persona that managed to transcend the leering, "smutty" characters of the burlesque hall. Mae West's famous "Is that a gun in your pocket?" innuendo has disappeared. What's left is simple sexuality.

It is hard to reconstruct the power of this gesture. In the 1950s popular culture still felt the repressive thrall of Victorian sexuality. It still believed sex was supposed to acknowledge its "depravity" with a smirk or a leer. In a culture of this sort, Marilyn's kind of sexuality was simply sensational. It was so perfectly generous, unqualified, accessible. Norman Mailer feels its effect still: "... Marilyn was deliverance, a very Stradivarius of sex, so gorgeous, forgiving, humorous, compliant and tender."[16]

The New Meanings of Blondness

The new self Monroe created in *Gentlemen Prefer Blondes* gave birth to a new kind of blondness. The new meanings of openness, access, transparency and the perfect gift that she invented for "Marilyn" took up residence in her hair. After Monroe, blondness came to stand for a sexual, emotional and intellectual openness. It came to stand for access of every kind. Once the colour of peek-a-boo, blondness was now the colour of full disclosure.

But inevitably, blondness also soaked up the unhappy side of Monroe's creation. After "Marilyn," blondness also came to stand for women who were unable to establish autonomy or defend the self. It became an invitation for the worst kinds of male attention. Blondness now stood for new kinds of openness and selflessness that were, willy-nilly, new kinds of vulnerability and subordination.

Some women have found a way to wear their blondness that accepts the good and avoids the bad. They are heirs to Marilyn's blondness, but not its captives. Modern Marilyns pick and choose their way through blondness, trying out what they like, refusing what they don't. Modern Marilyns exploit the powers of blondness selectively.

Susan Sarandon has used blondness to play out sexuality and emotional access. But she is not a passive recipient of the heritage. She takes care. She expresses a self that is sexually and emotionally accessible but bounded

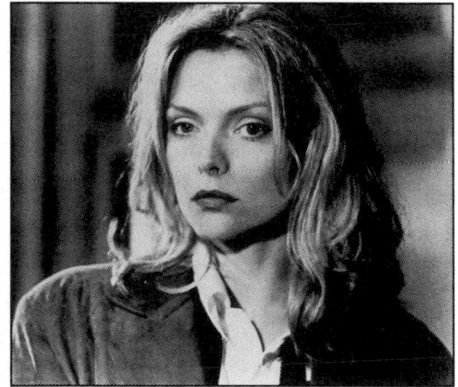

"Marilyn" blondness at will

and guarded as well. This modern Marilyn treats blondness as a repertoire of possibilities, some to be embraced, some to be avoided.

Other blondes demonstrate the ability to tap blondness without being claimed by it. Kathleen Turner, Ellen Barkin, Jessica Lange and Michele Pfeiffer all demonstrate that they can "do" Marilyn blondness at will. All four of them use it to show sexual and emotional access. These women are carefully selective about how they use the tradition.

Blondness After Marilyn: Linda Evangelista's Blond Moment

There was a sensation in 1990 when model Linda Evangelista suddenly dyed her brown hair blond. The *Women's Wear Daily* was especially nasty: "She was striking as a brunette, but as a blonde she looks, well, just ordinary."[17]

Linda Evangelista did not remain a blonde for long. In less than a year, she had moved on, first to red hair and then to black. When asked to explain these sudden shifts, Evangelista said: "I had blond hair for nine months. I did everything I wanted as a blond."[18]

Linda's blond moment

Evangelista is famous for this kind of versatility. Ronnie Cook, a creative director for the New York store Barneys, said recently, "She gets better with age or, like Madonna, keeps re-inventing herself. I really feel she had a different persona with us...."[19]

Evangelista believes she has a protean quality. As she

puts it, "I think my [portfolio] kills everybody's. Every time you turn the page, it's a different person."[20] She is constantly taking on new looks. Blondness was for her an experiment, a chance to try out the many meanings of blondness. Once Evangelista had "done everything she wanted" as a blonde, she moved on.

This marks a new attitude towards blondness and to hair colour in general. It marks the end of blondness as a lifelong commitment. Evangelista's approach is more playful. Blondness becomes a resource, an opportunity for self-exploration, one of many rest stops in the road to self-discovery.

For some women, the rewards of blondness are no longer enough

Modern Marilyns use Monroe's legacy with skill and care. They are pulling out of it the meanings that are useful and jettisoning the rest. They are discriminating in a way Monroe herself could not afford to be.

The Blonde Rebellion

Monroe's heritage is being refused outright by many women. Several natural blondes I talked to are sick and tired of their hair colour. One university student told me:

> When I am listening to a professor in a lecture hall, and she has long puffy blond hair, I hate it, but I have trouble giving her the same attention. It's been drilled into us that the dippy blond look is connected with low intelligence. Look at "Three's Company."

Some women have been persuaded that blondness is now a ghetto so filled with demeaning stereotypes that they do not want to live there any more.

But there are pay-offs to being a blonde, and it's hard to let them go. As one blonde put it, "People do things for you when you are blond. They give you things! They let you into traffic!" Another said, "People thought I was ditsy, a bimbo, and I think I might have played it up a bit. For some reason I liked the attention that acting kind of stupid got me."

For some women, the rewards of blondness are no longer enough. Increasingly, these women are blondes in revolt, women who are prepared to renounce the advantages, and cut or colour what was once their crowning glory.

Generally, they came to this by stages. The first is usually the recognition that men are attracted by blondness, not the person. Blondes are discovering, to their horror, that blondness is a Pavlovian signal *any* woman can use to attract *any* man. At this moment, their blondness ceases to be *their* blondness. As one woman told me, "My hair colour had nothing to do with me. It was kinda insulting. So I chopped it off."

The Madonna Story

Once the colour of femaleness in our culture, blondness is for some women the flag of a deeply compromised vision of what it is to be a woman. If blondness is to survive in our culture, it will need reinvention.

Madonna may be just the woman for the job. If she is Marilyn incarnate, it's not by accident. Madonna is well known for her debt to Marilyn Monroe. The video "Material Girl" is a deliberate imitation of Monroe and her "Diamonds Are a Girl's Best Friend" performance in *Gentlemen Prefer Blondes*.

Madonna borrowed the image of Marilyn only to reinvent it

Outspoken academic Camille Paglia resists the comparison. She claims there is no important resemblance between Madonna and Monroe.[21] To my mind, this is simply wrong, but let's grant Paglia this much: there are times when Madonna resembles Mae West as much as she does Marilyn Monroe. If Monroe took away the dance hall sexuality of blondness, Madonna appears to be putting it right back in. She has resurrected the dame, the gun moll. She has made her blondness exactly what she made it in the film *Dick Tracy*, a statement of gum-snapping, brazen self-sufficiency. Madonna has resurrected the blonde who wants to know if that's a gun in your pocket.

In a sense, this brings us full circle. The openness and accessibility Monroe created for her sexuality and blondness is drained away. We are left with something harder, more closed, more defended. We are left with a closing up of Marilyn's openness, with an armouring of the self.

Why would Madonna do such a thing? Why tinker with one of the great symbolic resources of our culture? The answer is simple. Madonna is looking for power. Mae West's blondness is a great way to claim high explosives. Monroe's blondness is too tame. Madonna has spotted the vulnerabilities of Monroe's heritage. She is refusing its powerlessness and vulnerability. The last thing Madonna wants is a vacant, unprotected self and the promise of access. Madonna refuses this kind of blondness.

What Madonna wants is a return to the oldest and the most sexist versions of femaleness. She

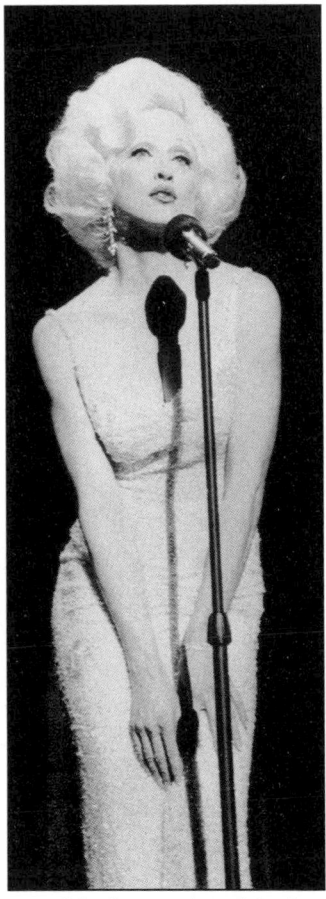

Madonna does Marilyn

wants the candour and the toughness of the vaudeville vamp. She wants the fully sexual, resourceful self-sufficiency of the Mae West character. And the stigma of the "bad girl"? Madonna just laughs it off. She is happy to use this stigma for effect, and just as happy to cast it aside as irrelevant. The bad girl stigma costs her nothing.

This is a complete rethinking of the Marilyn version of

sex and blondness. It dispenses with innocence, emotional access and the notion of sex as a gift. Madonna's Mae West sexuality (and blondness) is knowing, cunning, calculating. It is also toughened up, completely without vulnerability. As it turns out, Madonna borrowed the image of Marilyn only to reinvent it.

What has Madonna wrought? It is, I think, a little too early to tell. Some people are persuaded that Madonna has accomplished something of clear and lasting value. Camille Paglia applauds Madonna's accomplishment:

> Madonna has taught young women to be fully female and sexual while still exercising control over their lives. She shows girls how to be attractive, sensual, energetic, aggressive, ambitious and funny—all at the same time.[22]

Other people are less sure. They say Madonna does not transcend sexist stereotypes; they say she trades in them.

I am taking a bold and courageous position — up here on the fence. I think it depends on how well Madonna plays it out. If she succeeds in breaking open our stereotypes to recover the power inside, we are fine. Her adventure in the land of sexism will have been a stunning success. If, instead, Madonna rehabilitates the stereotypes of Mae West blondness, we're in real trouble. Madonna will have succeeded in calling up the most damaging and dangerous images of women, and she will have given them new credibility. There is a third possibility: that she will retreat from blondness altogether. In recent performances we have seen her appear with shades of brown and black.

Madonna *has* done something extraordinary. She may even be a cultural inventor of Marilyn Monroe's standing. If her experiment works, we will have a new version of sexuality and blondness, and a new architect of blondness. If it doesn't, Madonna will be our Icarus, another blonde who flew too near the sun.

Brunettes and Redheads:
The Rise of the Non-blonde

*A*ll the great beauties of the world are brunettes. It is brunettes who win hearts, stop tongues and take the breath away. It is brunettes who rule men's hearts. It is brunettes who make men cry.

That got your attention, didn't it? We are not accustomed to hearing brown hair praised. It is, usually, the residual colour, what you're left with if you don't move to blond, red or black. The stereotype says that brown hair is for people with no sense of drama, confidence or force of personality. It's for the timid, the meek and the mild.

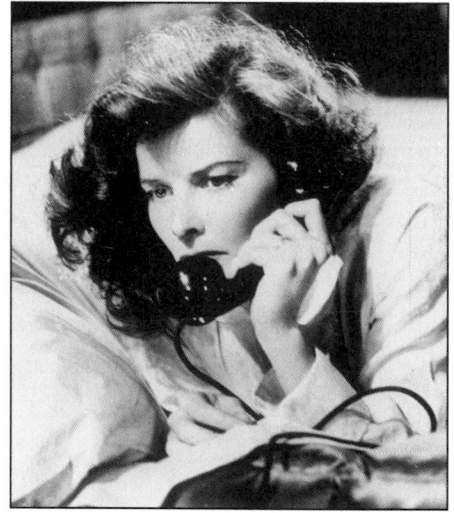

Katharine Hepburn: Stunning brunette

The time has come to speak more generously of brown hair. It is time to acknowledge its transformational powers.

Brown hair is the perfect complement to beauty. It is the real companion of self-confidence. Brown hair is the supporting cast that lets women claim centre stage. After all, women *wear* brown hair; it doesn't wear them.

Blond hair is, by contrast, a selfish colour. It seeks attention well, but it is frequently working on its own behalf. When a blonde creates a sensation in traffic, the wearer gets only *some* of the credit. Blondness takes the rest. Ask men what they saw. "Oh, well, a blonde," they will tell you, blinking at the sheer difficulty of the question. They didn't see the person. They saw a hair colour. They saw an icon. Hence the blonde's dilemma: "Is it me or my hair?"

> *Brown hair is an enabling colour. It enhances a woman's beauty without claiming to be her beauty.*

And what about the redhead? Red hair is a colour with powerful meanings that provokes powerful reactions. But often this is the hair talking, not the wearer.

Blond and red hair declare themselves at a distance, well before you can see the person wearing them. As they approach, all the stereotypes of the colour come rushing into consciousness. Finally, the wearer arrives, but by then it's too late. There is no room. Your mind is filled with all the conventional notions. The wearer is once more just a handy plinth, a medium for the message, a carrier of the colour, just another redhead.

Not brunettes! Brunettes carry no particular message. They are not slaves to any particular stereotype. They are not capsized by the meanings of their hair colour; the message never gets obscured by the medium. Brown hair does not compete with the wearer for attention. It is not selfish. It does not try to hog the limelight. Brown hair lets you see the wearer.

Brunettes do not announce themselves from a long way off—which lets them take you by surprise. A man is marching down the sidewalk, lost, perhaps, in thought. And suddenly, whammo! He's been claimed by a brunette. He aches for another glimpse, but she is gone. He has possessed beauty and lost it.

Brown hair is an enabling colour. It enhances a woman's beauty without claiming to *be* her beauty. It is left to the viewer to decide what this beauty is. Brown hair gives you no clue, no instruction, and it provides no interference.

This makes brown the "transformational" colour par excellence. It is, after all, all the colours combined. As one fashion journalist puts it, "One of the biggest shifts in thinking about brown is that the complexity of its color … is being recognized." She quotes Louis Licari, one of the great Manhattan colourists: "If you look at brunette hair, it's rarely all one shade. Medium-brown hair, for example, will have many different tones, from golden strands to dark brown, and there might be some red or sunburn in it, too.[1] Brown hair, far from being "mousy" and "drab," provides a wide palette of possibilities, all of which can be used to represent the diverse aspect of the brunette's self.

The brunette can be a hot beauty, or she can be a cool beauty. She can be a beauty of great refinement or of perfect sensuality. She can be ethereal or earthy, distant or vivid, exotic or familiar. The brunette can even be the mind-stopping combination of all these things. Brown hair creates possibilities, not obligations. For women

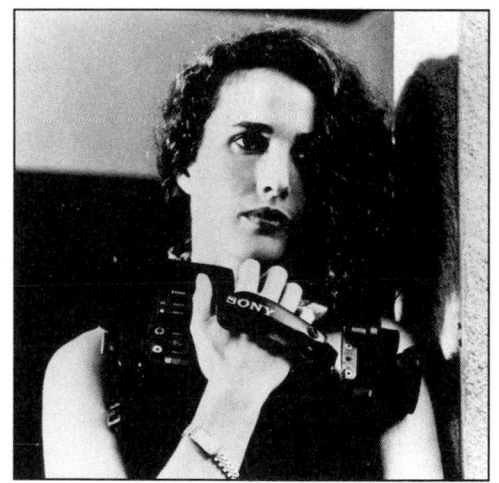

Andie MacDowell: The new brunette

who wish to make their own decisions about who they are, brown hair scores high.

Brown hair is especially powerful because it works so well with skin. Blond hair often washes women out. It is busy capturing and casting as much light as it can. The face that is not endowed with strong and vivid features loses out. Black hair on white women can create a terrible contrast between hair and skin, making the face pale and sallow by comparison. You have to have the big-featured beauty of an Anjelica Huston to survive the contrast (or be a blanche-faced Gothic who doesn't care).

Brown hair makes beautiful skin glow. It sets up a tension between the two that is neither competitive nor cruelly contrastive. Several movie stars have exploited this tension to very good effect. Some of the beauty of Andie MacDowell (*Sex, Lies and Videotape, Groundhog Day, Four Weddings and a Funeral*) comes from the play between her skin and her hair. Winona Ryder (*Mermaids, Edward Scissorhands, Reality Bites*) also has "second look" beauty of the first order. The more you look at her, the more her beauty manifests itself.

Brunettes can do sexuality with great discretion. They do effortlessly what the Hitchcockian blondes could do only by artifice. They can turn up the volume of their sexuality by carefully modulated degrees: unlike the blondes, who start loud and stay loud, brunettes reveal their sexuality in stages. Brunettes do not trumpet a sexual message, as some blondes and redheads do. Instead, the message steals up on you and takes you unawares.

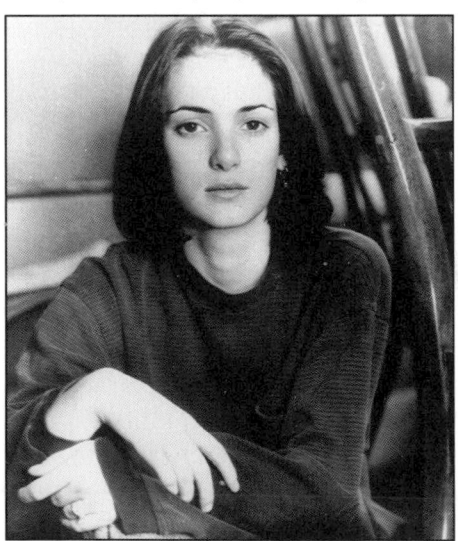

Winona Ryder: The new brunette

Traditionally, our opinion of brunettes has not been generous. People say this is the "blah" colour. "This is the colour you have if you don't have the sense to go blond or redhead," an older respondent told me. She complained brunettes were constantly being used in the 1980s ads for the professional working woman. "She always wore glasses and had this real serious expression on her face. It was, like, this one *must* have a brain, she's got brown hair!" Brown hair needs an image make-over by a public relations firm.

There was a time when brown hair was regarded as an unwelcome, even tragic, accident of birth

As the blond regime established itself in the '40s and '50s, Hollywood became increasingly unkind to brunettes. A quick tour of *Leonard Maltin's Movie and Video Guide* tells the story. From the 1930s onwards, there have been no fewer than twenty-six films celebrating blondness in their titles, including *Incendiary Blonde, Platinum Blonde, Adventurous Blonde* as well as *Blonde Trouble, Blonde Bait, Blonde Blackmailer, Blonde Crazy, Blonde Dynamite* and *Blonde Fever*. The "brunette" was so favoured exactly twice: *My Favorite Brunette* (1947) and *Gentlemen Marry Brunettes* (1955).

Hollywood, one of the great creators of our culture, has used brown hair over and over again to suggest a retiring personality, a lack of confidence, a certain unworldliness. Take the example of the otherwise forgettable movie *Superchick* (1973). This movie is about a blond flight attendant who is so pursued by men that she finally changes her hair colour to a mousy brown. Only then is she left alone. In this typical symbolism, blondness is the sign of excitement and glamour, and brunetteness, the ordinary and banal.

So much for Hollywood. What did the hair industry think about brunettes? Lawrence Gelb of Clairol, speaking in 1961, was unambiguous about it: "Nine out of ten women would choose to be blondes if they could do it by pressing a button. Nothing ever has induced women to favor dark hair."[2] Naturally, Gelb had a vested interest. Clairol was selling a lot of bottled blondness at the time. But he's right, there was a time when brown was not a colour anyone chose. There was a time when brown hair was regarded as an unwelcome, even tragic, accident of birth.

You can blame most of this on Marilyn Monroe. It was she, as we have seen, who legitimized the blonde. After Monroe, blond could be both sexy *and* innocent. Brown hair was now truly eclipsed. It had become the mark of domesticity, wifeliness and a certain absence of personality. There were good qualities to all of this, to be sure. But when it came to winning the hearts of men, brown hair didn't do it. As one commentator observed:

> A psychiatrist once wrote (unfortunately) that blondes are the ones men like to date, brunettes are the ones men marry. And somehow it stuck. He said brunettes are warm, intelligent, romantic, down-to-earth, steadfast, faithful—I mean, it's enough to make you sick![3]

Brown Hair: The New Look

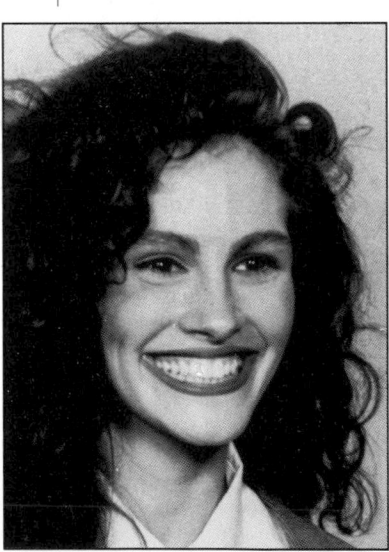

Julia Roberts: The new brunette

Fortunately, the world may be changing. Brown hair appears to be undergoing a transformation. As the 1990s started, we heard journalists summoning a laudatory language for brown hair. Now it's "shiny auburn, silky black-brown and rich chestnut."[4] Logan struck a blow for reevaluation of the brunette when she declared "dark hair is now the most exciting, confident color in town."[5] Collier, in an article entitled "Bold Brunette" in *Glamour* magazine announced, "Blondes may always have fun, but brunettes—lustrous and chocolaty—are making the big beauty news now."[6]

Colourists have joined the movement. They no longer advise women to move away from brown hair. Louis Licari is clear on this point: "If you're a brunette, just be a great brunette. Who am I to tell people to go blond?"[7] These days, colourists say stay put.[8]

Part of this is being driven by the '90s feeling for naturalism. As *Vogue* describes it:

> Women used to put a lot of energy into trying to look completely different. Just as we've moved away from makeup designed to alter a woman's natural skin tone, so we are getting away from the artificial in hair color.[9]

More and more people are nervous about the many artificial substances in our lives. They look askance on colours that do not ring true. Brown is, by this reckoning, the *natural* colour.

Even Hollywood is coming around. It is now possible to be both a brunette and a starlet, as the likes of Sean Young demonstrate. And brunette continues to be the colour of choice for some of the established stars of the day. No one was impressed when Geena Davis and Julia Roberts moved to blondness, and they soon moved back.

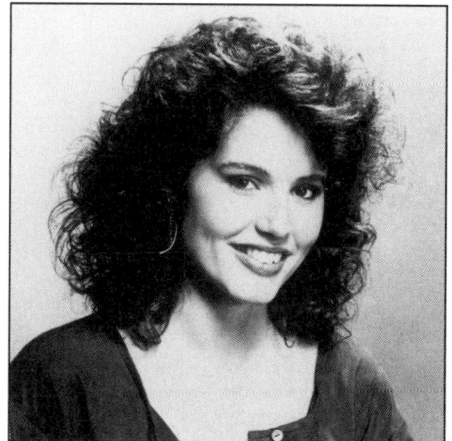

Geena Davis: The new brunette

Could any colour be better for the likes of Demi Moore? What colour becomes a woman of her beauty, intelligence and ability? Well, she tried blondness and then gave it up. Could she be a redhead? Unthinkable. How about hair as dark as Cher's? Impossible. Brown was the inevitable choice. Could it become the colour of choice for Hollywood's most powerful women?

As women continue to reclaim the self, brown hair will come into its own. As they continue to refuse sexist stereotypes and expectations of parents, husbands and children, brown looks better and better. It has no heritage of compromise. It has never been the colour you wear to please your man, the boss or a sexist male society. It has never been the plaything of Hollywood. It is a colour women can wear for themselves.

The patron saint of the brunette world is clearly the Hollywood star Joan Bennett. Bennett started her career as a blond ingenue in movies like *Little Women* (1933), but then she came to her senses. She returned to her natural, glossy brunette colour and rose to become one of the great stars of her time in *Man Hunt* (1941) and *Secret Beyond the Door* (1948).

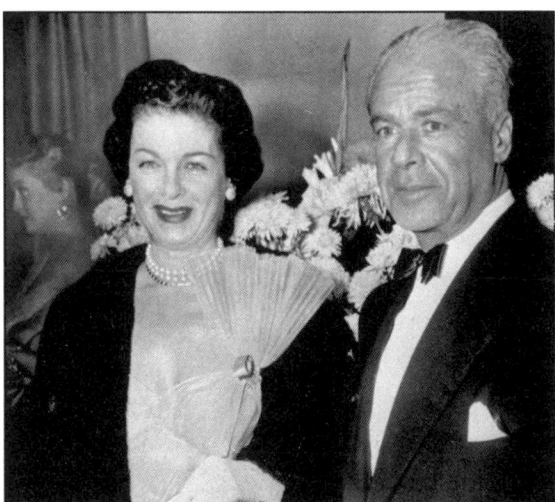

Joan Bennett: The patron saint of the brunette

How We Invented the Redhead: (A Letter of Apology)

In our society, we're not quite sure what red hair stands for, but we're pretty sure it means trouble. We associate red hair with mischief, stubbornness, temper, unpredictability and paradoxically both a certain strength and weakness of character. These are *not* the most sought-after qualities in our culture. They are not the ones that necessarily win you happiness at home or advancement in the world. Redheads alarm us a little. All that hair. All that colour. It's like a flag of warning: "Here comes trouble."

Surely someone with red hair like this must be some kind of anarchist

Red hair stands, in our culture, for temperamental qualities. It is Rita Hayworth in *Gilda*: controlled commotion. To be fair, red hair isn't about open hostility or aggression, but it does have a subtle, more social quality of menace. Redheads may not mean us any harm, exactly, but we take one look at their hair and wonder, "Will they be accommodating? Will they be agreeable?" Somewhere deep inside us, a little voice asks, "Surely someone with red hair like this must be some kind of anarchist."

Red hair stands for that mood we all feel sometimes: restless, irreverent, disinclined to do the right thing, delighted by the opportunity for mischief, eager to thumb our nose at authority and break the small rules of social conduct. If hair changed colour with our emotions, surely this is the colour it would turn when our patience was tested or our irreverence got the better of us. Or so we think. Redheads make us nervous because we imagine them ready to give vent to what we keep harnessed. Redheads are what we would be if we could do what we wanted to. Redheads represent our reckless, hot-headed, unconstrained side. After all, clowns have red hair. Clarabelle of the "Howdy-Doody" show had red hair. So does Homey, the bad-tempered clown on "In Living Color." It's hard to buy a fright wig that isn't red.

Redheaded children, we say, are inclined to mischief, and it turns out, in fact, that a disproportionate number of them are hyperactive.[10] There may be some natural, biological connection here. Or it may be that our stereotypes tell us that redheaded children should buzz with manic energy. We treat them accordingly and they oblige us.

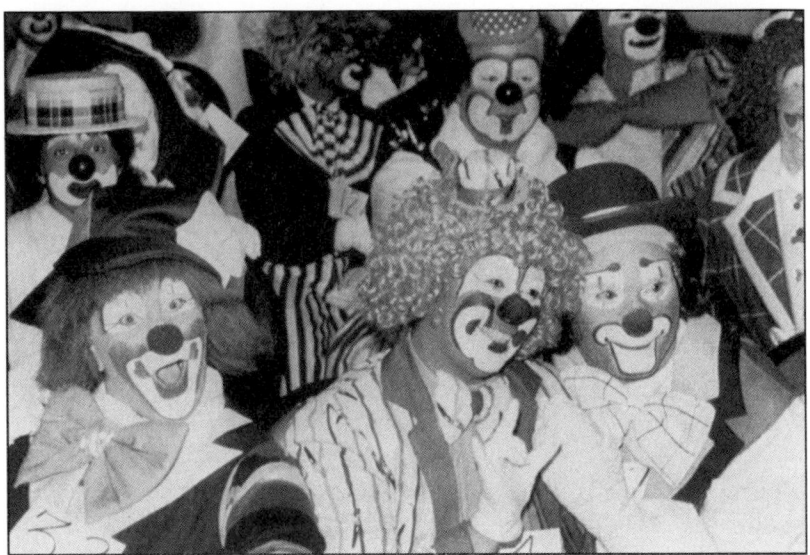

Red fright-wig hair

Nonconformity is another quality that is said to belong particularly to the redhead. We believe that redheads are wilful. Somehow we believe that people choose to spring from the womb with red hair. We see this astonishing and unlikely colour as a deliberate act of outrage. "If they refuse to conform in this," we say to ourselves a little nervously, "are they likely to conform in anything else?" We have our doubts. As one redhead told me, "People think my hair is such a statement. It's really just my hair."

We attribute stubbornness to the redhead. But why? We see lots of stubborn people in our lifetimes, and we make no connection between their hair colour and their mood. We have seen blondes in a snit and brunettes in a lather. But when someone has red hair, the stubbornness seems somehow inevitable. "Of course," we say to ourselves, "with hair like that, what do you expect but an outburst?"

The popular idea of Queen Elizabeth I plays this out. We have made her an icon of defiance. She would not budge for a favourite courtier, a crown prince or a representative of God. This is supposed to follow from her hair colour. Its redness declaimed a force of character that made her incapable of compromise.

Temper is also the mark of the redhead. We expect them to "go off." Proof? Well, we don't have any, really. Except there is something combustible about that hair. We speak of it as "flaming," in the same way we speak of tempers. We say, for example, "Rage consumed him, "He had to wait until his anger burned itself out," "His temper suddenly ignited." In our culture, both tempers and red hair are incendiary. Perhaps their association was inevitable.

One of the bombs dropped on Japan in World War II was named for the redheaded character Rita Hayworth played in *Gilda*. It's a telling piece of metaphor. Both the redhead and the bomb were seen to be explosive. (This is, incidentally, the origin of the "blonde bombshell" tag: after Marilyn Monroe, people decided blondes were even more incendiary than redheads.)

Strangely, we also have two contradictory views of the redhead. We believe that redheads have special powers of character or, alternatively, no real powers of character at all. On the one hand, they have a feeling for spontaneity and commotion the rest of us lack. They can marshal energies and a determination the rest of us cannot. On the other, we believe they are pulled helplessly behind runaway impulses, incapable of self-control.

Is there a pattern in all of this? Is it possible to

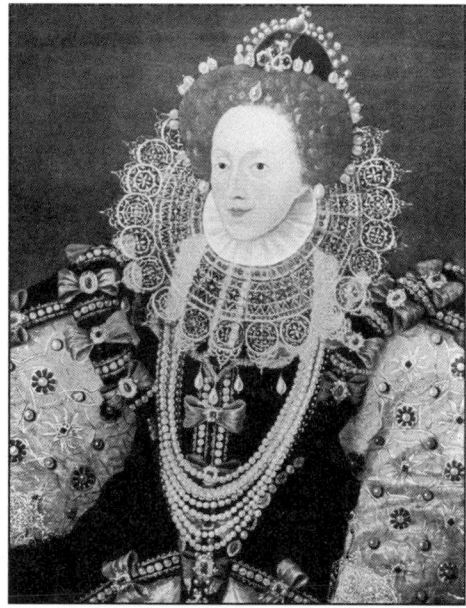

Queen Elizabeth I: In all her glory

make sense of it all? There is, I think, a cultural logic that makes our view of the redhead make sense. It has five easy pieces.

First, redheads make up just two percent of the population.[11] This is awkward. There are just enough of them that they cannot be classified as freaks, but so few of them that we never really get used to them. They are always exceptional. And being exceptional, they defy our categories. They are, in the language of anthropology, "liminal," on the margin, not quite fish and not quite fowl.

If only there were fewer of them. We could treat them as albino, as mistaken acts of nature, and have done with it. Or if only there were more of them. Then we could create a place for them and they would join blondes, brunettes and those with black hair as an expected and routine presence in our lives. As it is, redheads are too numerous to be ignored and too rare to be accepted.

> *Surely, we suppose, the colour of the hair is the temperature of the soul*

Second, redheads are easy targets. Because they are unexpected and unaccepted, we indulge our worst tendency. We do what humans always do when they find themselves in the presence of someone "different:" we begin to harbour unkind thoughts and stigmatizing suspicions. Surely, we suppose, the colour of the hair is the temperature of the soul. It tells us that this person is teeming with vivid, uncontrolled emotions that will spring from them as their hair does, unmediated, uncontrolled, somehow volcanic.

Third, redheads invite exile. We have made them exceptional and "different." We have invented an explanation for their difference: they are hot and dangerous. This next step is inevitable. Now we cast them out. Now we make them a scapegoat, load them up with our fears of mischief, stubbornness, temper and unpredictability, walk them to the edge of the village and send them trotting off into the night.

And the stigmatizing works! Studies show that men and women with red hair are "strongly disliked."[12] Redheaded men are especially loathed. One study advised men not to colour their hair red unless they want to "project the image of a comedian or of an antisocial person."[13] But it gets worse. A third study found that redheaded males were seen as "very unattractive, less successful, and rather effeminate." Older male redheads are particularly disliked. They are seen to be "sad, feminine, unpleasant, weak, slow and shallow"![14]

We are not quite so hard on redheaded women, but the hostility is still there. Redheaded women are seen to be untrustworthy and violent. There was a time when redheaded women were vilified as witches and burned at the stake.[15] Another of our favourite "casting out" strategies is to claim that redheads are not quite female. In childhood we call them tomboys. This is another way of saying that we cannot rely on them to embrace stereotyped qualities of femaleness, sweetness, docility and politeness. Redheads have not, until very recently, been sought after as fashion models, and this tells us just how far they are from the exemplars of femaleness in our culture.[16] Instead, we have seen them as wilful, irascible, impulsive, high-spirited. We respond with exile.

There is just one exception to this process of exclusion. We find redheaded children of both sexes endearing.[17] Anne Shirley, of the *Anne of Green Gables* books, is one of the most beloved of fictional children, in large part because of her spirited, redheaded personality. I was a redhead as a little boy, and the world forgave me everything, including bus fare, broken windows and bad manners. Red hair on a little boy is, according to the symbolic economy of our culture, threat plus non-threat. We have a name for this: it's called "cute." We are always charmed when the threatening is reduced. It fills us with relief and gratitude.

So there it is. Having loaded redheads up with all the qualities we fear in ourselves, we declare them dangerous;

having made them dangerous, we cast them out.

One last step left. Now that we have cast the redhead out, it is time to bring her back. As a lightning rod for our hostility, she is much too useful to be got rid of. We can ridicule in her what we fear in ourselves. All those frightening qualities now have a handy container, a place for safekeeping. We end the exile and readmit the redhead.

By this time, red hair has two opposing qualities: appeal and danger. Who is this creature that can summon stubbornness and wilfulness, who can rage with temper, who can change course, who is so little socialized that she can escape the rules and regulations that constrain the rest of us? We are attracted and repulsed.

Part of this fascination is sexual. Men are simultaneously alarmed but intrigued by redheaded women. Could they have special powers of sensuality? Their hair says that they have lively emotions, that they are unconstrained, that they are vivid and present. Is this an indication of the sexual character within?

Redheaded women send a double signal to men. They seem, on the one hand, to be disinclined to play out traditional gender roles or to act the perfect little companion. On the other hand, they promise sensual delights of extraordinary proportions. Perhaps this is why male writers like Tom Robbins have suggested that the redhead has an aura of "loveliness and danger."[18]

Another way we recover the banished redhead is by inviting her to play the trickster. In fact, we find her incendiary qualities intriguing. In small doses, we love them and cannot live without them. And we have so removed them from ourselves that we especially like them in someone else — particularly when this someone is a person we have stigmatized and can repudiate at will.

We like clowns, people who are not fully constrained by the rules of everyday life. And we especially like this mischief to come from people we can make fun of. If someone is going to make fun of us, we want to be able to make fun of them back. Clowns are perfect. They laugh at us; we laugh at them. Release and criticism is allowed but contained.

Five steps and the redhead is captured, identified, vested with meaning, cast out and returned to our midst. We have seized a colour and made it a symbol.

Red Hair as a Power Look

Lately, people have started to think about red hair a little differently. Some are even calling it a power look. In fact, there have always been women who wore their hair as a symbol of strength and character, who have played the "defiant redhead." People were quick to think of them as mischievous and stubborn, but these women didn't mind. Red hair gave them permission to have qualities women were normally denied. Red hair let you play the trickster. Red hair gave you powers you couldn't get any other way.

The rehabilitation of red hair takes us a step further. Now women are taking all the old qualities and reclaiming them. They are saying red hair stands for liveliness (not mischief), originality (not nonconformity), determination

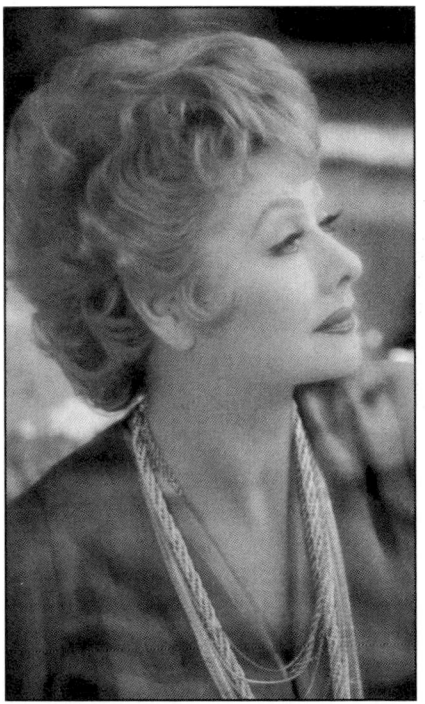

Lucille Ball: The archetypal redhead

(not stubbornness), passion (not temper), inventiveness (not unpredictability) and a decided (not dangerous) strength of character. Red hair is being charged with positive qualities.

In the words of one Toronto hairdresser: "Red hair? It's a real 'don't mess with me' colour."[19]

The stigmatizing treatment of the redhead charged it with some pretty formidable qualities. It took only a little bit of reengineering to release these qualities from the negative stereotype. Red hair may have had a troubled past, but this is what makes it so potent in the present day.

Redheads have come a very long way. No less a figure than Lacey Ford, a power in the modelling world, likes redheads. "A redhaired model," she suggested, "may make a stronger statement than a blonde or brunette."[20] The redhead has gone from being lovely but dangerous to being lovely because dangerous. It is now one of the colours that bespeaks resourcefulness, ambition and power. By the late '80s, things were changing. As *Harper's Bazaar* proclaimed, "Psychologists agree that the redhead look suggests a woman who's sure of herself and in charge of her life."[21]

By 1987, some five million women in the United States were keeping or choosing red hair.[22] These included stars, essential recruits in any war against obscurity, among them the rock star Lady Miss Kier and film star Nicole Kidman. Red hair is even finding its way into polite society: society doyenne Cornelia Guest switched from blond to red hair in 1988, as did Norris Church Mailer and Pat Lawford.

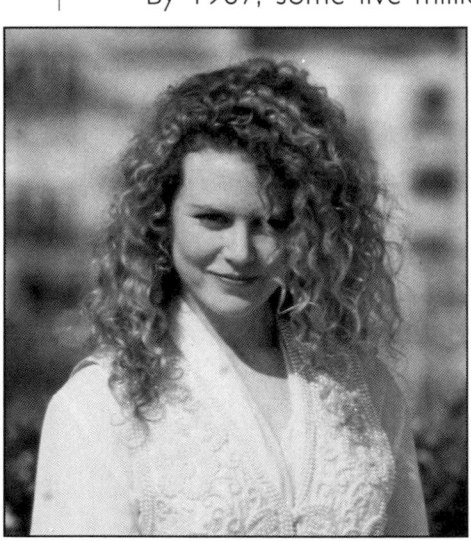

Nicole Kidman: Red hair for the '90s

The fashion press began to look kindly on red hair, and this is the most important "moral victory" for any hair colour that wishes to move up in the world. In 1988, Linda Wells of the *New*

York Times declared in an article entitled "Red is right now": "A year ago, blond was the color of the moment. This summer, those who were born red are flaunting it, and those who were not are giving nature a nudge."[23] Industry, the last and final frontier, has responded by introducing new shades of red. In 1970, L'Oréal had two shades. By 1989, they had sixteen, while Redken had twenty-nine shades and Clairol some forty-three.[24]

The danger of red hair has been harnessed as an advantage. *Harper's Bazaar*'s "Redhead Beauty Guide" declared in 1987: "Red hair now suggests someone who is sure of herself, is in charge of her own life and is proud of her sex and sexuality. After all, red means Danger! Fire! Risk!"[25]

"After all." As if this were the most natural association in the world. Red hair has come a long way in the last few years. What used to be dangerous and therefore bad is now dangerous and therefore good.

Georgette Mosbacher: Redhead Extraordinaire

Red hair is perfect for self-invention, a potent symbol for the redefinition of the social self. There cannot be a better example of this than that of Georgette Mosbacher, CEO of Georgette Mosbacher Enterprises and the former CEO of La Prairie. She is well known in Washington social circles, where she and her husband are a conspicuous presense.

Ms. Mosbacher has come a long way. She grew up in a steel town in Indiana, where she was a hairdresser in her youth. She has had to change shape dramatically in order to find her way to Washington, wealth and power. I have no doubt that being a hairdresser helped in all of this. It gave her a first-hand knowledge of the symbolic materials at her disposal. And it gave her an intimate acquaintance with the power of hair in the process of self-transformation. As she puts it, "I've certainly reinvented myself on numerous occasions."

Ms. Mosbacher chose red hair carefully.

I was just out of college when I said, "OK, Georgette, this is the defining moment. You're going out there. Here are your goals. Let's go get them." I wasn't born with flaming red hair, but I knew that I was born to have it. I've been called "the most determined redhead since Moll Flanders."

"Defining moment," is, for our purposes, a perfect choice of words. Like Marilyn Monroe, Ms. Mosbacher has had to resist the definitional efforts of others. In Washington, the press does not hesitate to assign roles. Ms. Mosbacher's husband is invariably called a CEO while she is cast as the "socialite" and a "trophy wife."

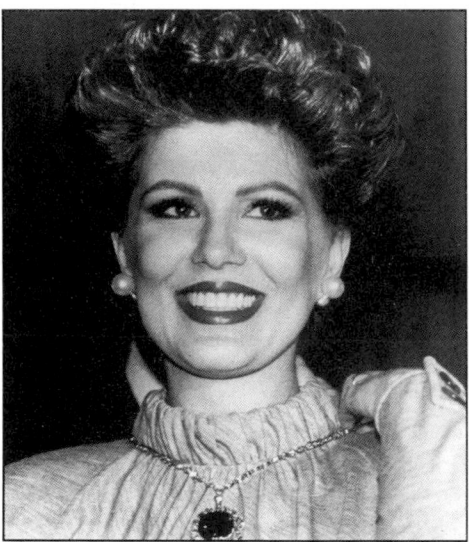

Georgette Mosbacher: The most determined redhead since Moll Flanders

What really serves Ms. Mosbacher in her attempt to claim a non-ornamental place in Washington life is that very red hair. Wham! It gives fair warning. This is not the colour of deference, dependency or submission. This hair says "Take me seriously or leave me alone."[26]

Rita Hayworth, Patron Saint of the Redhead

If Joan Bennett is the patron saint of the brunette set and Marilyn Monroe the patron saint of blondes, there can be no question that Rita Hayworth is patron saint of the redheads. Hayworth began her career as a Spanish beauty (she was born Margarita Carmen Dolores Cansino) with dark hair. The studio, in its wisdom, decided something had to be done. Helen Hunt, the chief hairstylist at Columbia, recommended a switch to auburn and electrolysis to correct a low hairline. Red hair became Hayworth's trademark and a symbol for her considerable accomplishments as a dancer, actress and star.[27]

Hayworth then had the misfortune to marry Orson Welles. Actually, it was worse than that. Hayworth made Welles her husband and then she made him her director. Jealous of her fame, Welles proved possessive on the first count and dictatorial on the second. For *The Lady from Shanghai* (1948), he insisted Hayworth cut her hair short and colour it blond. He even supervised while the deed was done.[28]

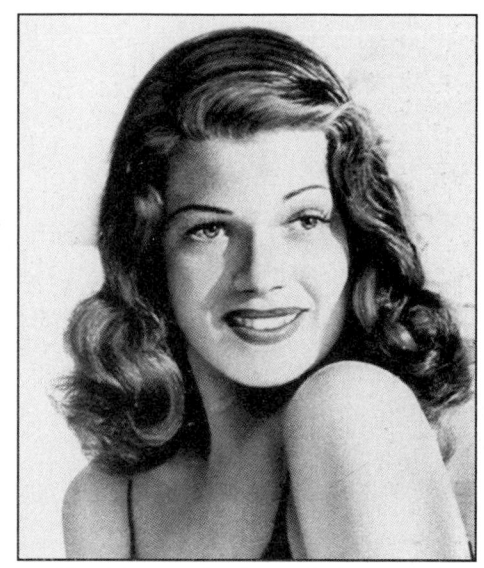

This was a ruthless bit of manipulation. It stripped Hayworth of the colour that had been one of the most useful instruments and symbols of her ascendancy. Hayworth soon divorced her power-seeking husband. She returned to red hair and her own identity.

What began as the colour of children, comics and clowns is now a flag of determination. Jill, one of my interviewees, is a

Rita Hayworth: Controlled commotion

redhead, and she has a redheaded daughter of eleven. As a girl, Jill hated red hair. She wanted to blend in, and her hair would not let her. Whether she liked it or not, she was marked as different.

And different, it turns out, attracts different. Not so long ago, Jill was sitting on the subway when a man pulled out a guitar and started singing her Gene Autry songs. When she asked him what he thought he was doing, he replied, "I just love your hair."

Adding Colour and Going Grey:
How Colour Transforms

No woman should be allowed near a bottle of
bleach. It's like feeding whisky to the Indians. She
doesn't know when to stop. She starts out intend-
ing to lighten her hair just a shade, but within a
week she imagines herself as a golden-haired child
and winds up looking like something out of a
chamber of horrors."

Charles Revson, 1961 [1]

Generally speaking, men regard the colouring of hair
with the same suspicion and alarm that they have
brought to everything in the world of hair. It's another
instrument of magic they do not understand. Their
response has been dismissive (and, in Revson's case, sexist
and racist). They have belittled hair colouring and mocked
the women who have used it.

Women feel differently. Colouring hair is one of the
great instruments of self-transformation in their lives.
Speaking in the early 1960s, an industry professional said:

All women go through a period when they'd like to
have different personalities and changing the color of

their hair is the quickest way to do it. That's particularly true after an emotional crisis. The best prospects
for coloring are divorcees and young widows.[2]

But men's opinion of colouring has generally won out.
Until quite recently, colouring was a guilty secret never to
be revealed. In 1961 Mrs. Iris Goodman, of Antoine de
Paris beauty salons, said, "None of us old-timers
in the field ever thought we'd hear hair coloring
mentioned in polite company…. Women used
to be so sensitive that they never asked for a
coloring job; they wanted a 'treatment.'"[3]

Colouring was
a guilty secret

Some women created a pretext for hair
colour. They claimed to have suffered an emotional shock
that turned their hair white. They needed a "treatment" to
return things to normal. Naturally, no one in the salon ever
believed a word of this, but it was a delicate, discreet way
for women to ask for something that, strictly speaking, they
were not entitled to.

Colouring was a guilty secret for many reasons. First, it
was something only "fast" women were supposed to do. It
was, in the Jean Harlow / Mae West model, the mark of a
woman who had lax morals and who used her badge of
promiscuity to prey on the defenceless husbands of other
women. It was a sign of sexual and moral impropriety.

Furthermore, colouring was often seen as "lower
class," because it was frequently obvious, the
first error of all status misconduct. And it occa-
sioned the punishment that is visited on anyone who misbehaved in this way: status loss.
Colouring your hair could cost you both your
moral and your social standing.

She was a
"bottle blonde"

But the shame of colouring went deeper than this,
right down into the very foundations of the sexism of our
culture. Men want women to look a certain way, but they
want them to look that way "naturally." When men discover that women have *worked* to make themselves conform

to their expectations, all bets are off. These women are "cheating." They are resorting to deception. In the case of hair colour, it's a classic double-bind. Women who were going grey had to resort to colouring if they wanted male attention, but if they were found out, male attention was withdrawn. Not surprisingly, they took refuge in secret codes. "Treatments" were the order of the day.

Women could be just as harsh as men. If they discovered that another woman had coloured her hair, they would happily use it against her. In the war of every woman against every woman in 1950s America, one of the most effective ways to crush a competitor was to quietly let slip that she was a "bottle blonde." There were few better ways of calling her morality into question. She was, after all, cheating at the dating game. She was resorting to false advantages. And she was misrepresenting herself on the marriage market, where every

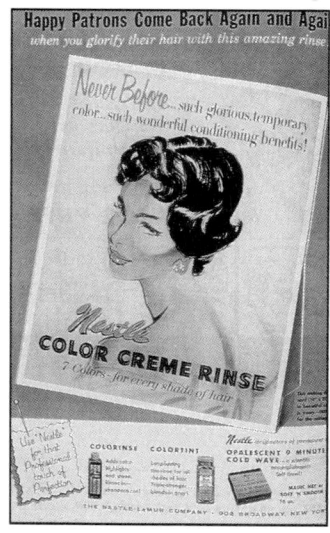

man sought honesty and uprightness in the potential mother of his children.

None of this was lost on Lawrence Gelb, president of Clairol. Gelb brought back a revolutionary new colouring technology from Europe in 1931. It was revolutionary because it reduced the colouring time from hours to minutes and, most important, it could be performed at home. But the real cunning of the new product was linguistic. Gelb insisted

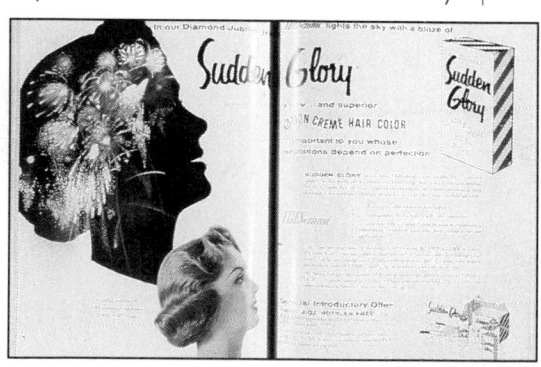

that his new product was not a "dye." It was, he said, a "tint." American women sighed with relief and began, tentatively and with care, to adopt this once scandalous, still exotic practice.

By 1950, *Life* magazine estimated that some ten million American women were using dye, and the magazine was prepared to say that "dyed hair…no longer automatically labels a woman as 'fast.'"[4] You can see a shadow of disapproval here still. But the following year, *Life* appeared to have softened even further. The magazine was now advocating a metal powder as a means of temporarily tinting the hair, a powder "derived from the aluminum dust inhaled by miners to coat their lungs as protection from coal gas." One of science's little treasures, to be sure, and a horror to our modern, Alzheimer's-anxious ears.[5] This was progress in one area, but not in another. The social risks of hair treatment were going down. The health risks were not.

By 1953, *Vogue* was claiming, without any evidence or a shred of plausibility, that virtually every American woman had "toyed" with hair colouring. This was plainly an exaggerated claim but it shows that some publications were well beyond the fear of colouring.[6] By 1957, *Look* noted approvingly that fifty-five million American women were adding colour to their hair. The article shows "before" and "after" shots for several women. The "after" shots show them basking in their husbands' approval.[7] The sexism of these photos is irritating, but they suggest that men were being encouraged to accept the colouring practice. The guilty secret was now less guilty and less secret.

Nevertheless, that old tone of censure was still very much in circulation. In 1961 Stanley Frank declared, with a trace too much emphasis, that it was no longer "only actresses and women of dubious character [who] flaunted dyed hair."[8] The odour of disapproval is still detectable. The next year, flight attendants were forced to fight for the right to colour their hair. The airlines would not budge. Sounding for all the world like dear old Judge Lomenzo, an airline executive warned the nation of terrible consequences: "If you let those girls run wild there's no telling what would happen. They might end up with green hair to match the seat coverings."[9]

The 1960s was a crucial decade for these attitudes, as it was for so many others. In 1963, *Newsweek* was at last able to talk about hair colour without a trace of condescension or discomfort: "Does she or doesn't she? The answer is yes, she does."[10] The guilty secret was out of the closet. By the end of the 1960s, there were reported to be ten manufacturers of dye in the United States.[11] Women no longer asked covertly for "treatments." Hair colour was increasingly a fact of life.

Hair colour continued to grow in respectability through the 1970s, and by 1981, things had really changed. To quote Georgia Dullea in the *New York Times*: "Clearly, the question 'Does she or doesn't she?' has become irrelevant. The question now posed by the sight of a gray-haired woman...is: 'Why doesn't she?'[12]

By the 1990s, the stigma attached to colouring one's hair had completely disappeared. According to *Vogue*, in 1988, American women were spending a staggering 3.3 billion dollars for hair colouring services and products.[13] *Working Woman* magazine estimated in 1992 that 40 percent of American women coloured their hair.[14] This figure is almost certainly conservative. *Vogue*'s early estimate has come to pass. Now it seems likely that most women in America have experimented with colour, and the majority of them use it routinely.

Colourists: A New Profession

Another measure of colouring's new respectability is that by the 1980s it had created its own profession: the colourist. And a good thing, too. There were by the early '90s nearly five hundred shade names for blonds and a really good colourist will use some twenty of them at a time.[15] Colouring was being systematized. The art was becoming a science and the science an art. To manage the endless possibilities before them, colourists invented a new language: bloops, ribbons, flashes, skimming, misting, match-lites and spiral lights.[16] The profession had arrived.

The profession of colourists was established in the '60s. By the '90s, in the time-honoured tradition of the profession, they were declaring themselves "artists."[17] As usual, this metaphor does not serve especially well. This is, after all, a group who routinely transform millions of people. Artists have dreamed of this role in the life of popular culture but have never come close to achieving it. Surely, colourists deserve better!

Women use colour to say goodbye to old selves and to audition new ones

What Is Colour For?

In our guiltless era, people use colour to transform themselves. Women use it to look older and to look younger. They use it to make themselves look softer and more gracious and they use it to make themselves look more forthright and formidable. They use colour to declare the end of one relationship and they use it to open up the possibility of others. Women use colour to say goodbye to old selves and they use it to audition new ones.

Some women use hair colour to help them claim maturity and to get on with life.

> Going blond changed my life. It was the summer of 1966. I was fifteen. I was at the cottage and I felt overweight and really unattractive. To make matters worse, my sister was older than me and extremely popular. So one night I got a bottle of peroxide and bleached my hair. I thought I looked very glamorous. The boys did too.

This is hair colouring at its most basic. Just a girl with a bottle of chemicals and a plan. It's a long way from the genius of New York colourist Oribe in a salon filled with the latest technology in the world of hair colour. But the effect is not altogether different. This young woman used hair colour to raise the flag of sexual intent. The world paid attention. The transformation started. She was, as she put it, "never the same. It just changed the way I thought about myself."

Hair colour can be used to contend with racial stereotypes. One of my respondents told me that these days her Chinese friends are adding blondness to their hair. "They do it so people will think they are Filipinos. Filipinos are the party animals of Asia, the ones with personality. They want to look like someone with personality."

Ours is a culture that has ceased to offer a standard "coming of age" ritual. It is not, as the professional lamenters like to claim, because we are a culture that has lost touch with itself and its own tradition. It is because there is no longer a single notion of womanhood towards which all girls are headed. In our culture, there are literally dozens of versions of femaleness. No ritual could possibly deliver young girls to all of these new gender stations. So we leave rites of passage to the individual. It is she who must decide who she wants to become and how she wants to get there. Hair colouring can be part of this critical self-assertion.

Colour is also used to fight advancing age. There is a notion that blondness in particular helps to soften the appearance of an ageing woman, that it softens the play of light around her face, that it diminishes the effect of wrinkles and lines. Some women even treat colouring as a substitute for plastic surgery. They claim, rightly or wrongly, that a good colourist can take years off your age.

This addition of colour is made more urgent by the effects of age upon hair itself. There is, in the words of Wilma F. Bergfeld, M.D., a "poop out" factor for hair. As it ages, hair loses its shine and volume. Richard Hudavoni, of the Rocco and Altobelli Salon in Minneapolis, observes,

"Blond hair fades and becomes more 'opaque,' brunettes lose their natural gold or auburn highlights, and reds just brown out."[18] Colour not only replaces shine, it also adds volume.

There are dangers here, of course. Women who resort to blondness to soften their appearance often keep right on going and end up too blond. It's easy to make this transition. The eye gets accustomed to the new blondness of your hair and you add more to get the same effect. This is roughly the same thing as overdoing perfume. And it is not only women who are guilty of this. As Pauline Kael once said of Robert Redford, "He has turned almost alarmingly blond — he's gone past platinum, he must be plutonium; his hair is coordinated with his teeth."[19]

But not everyone moves to blondness. Diana Vreeland is a famous example of *renewed* black hair. As a master in the language of fashion, she knew what black hair could do for her, and in her imperial manner she ordered it done. Punks and Goths are also inclined to colour their hair black. They do this for the same reason Vreeland did: to tell the world they are creatures to be reckoned with.

One of my respondents, Carol, told me how she used hair colouring when she began teaching in the 1980s at Bodger Preparatory Day, an old and conservative private school on the eastern seaboard. Carol had gone to the school as a girl, and she knew she needed some way to keep herself from being swallowed by what she calls "the Bodger myth." She needed an "edge." Her solution: electric streaks of neon colour in her hair.

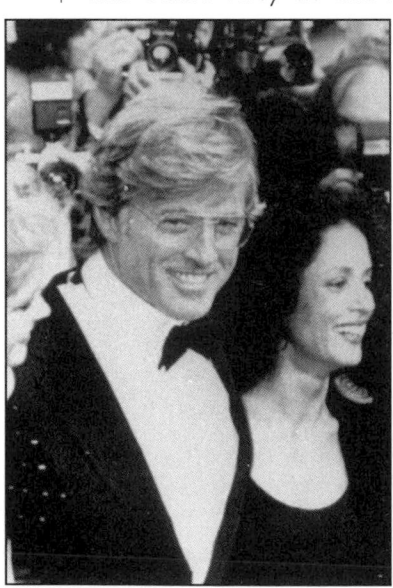

Robert Redford: Plutonium Blonde

The administrators at Bodger's did double-takes hard enough to get whiplash. After all, this was a WASP institution devoted to discretion in everything, especially self-presentation. Bodger's teaches young girls, among other things, the arts of discretion and the secret codes of status. Carol's electric hair flew in the face of all of that. It looked, one matron said, like Carol's hair was on fire. It looked, said one delighted student, like she had been captured by fairies, carried across dew-damp college lawns in the first light of day and festooned with whimsical colours. Carol's hair was a contradiction of just about everything Bodger's stood for.

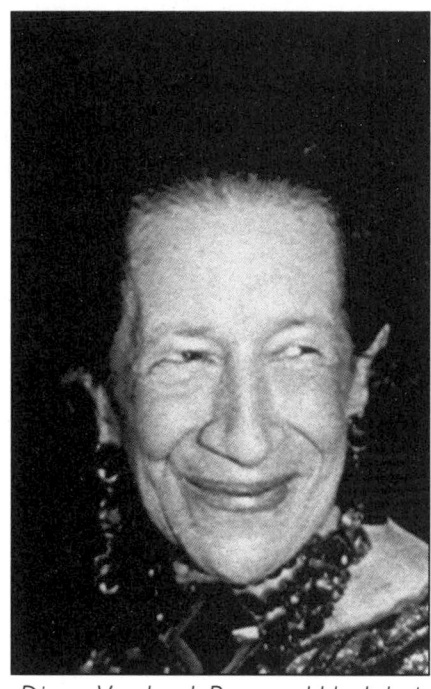

Diana Vreeland: Renewed black hair

Needless to say, the students loved it. Carol came to represent the exotic new world out there, the world they would some day enter after they left "the nunnery." And, strangely, even the administrators came to love it. Carol's hair became their little act of bravery, their one slightly thrilling, slightly terrifying acknowledgment of the "modern" world. The bravest of them came to see Carol's hair as a sign of the new breed of thoroughly modern Bodger girl. Carol became their pet, their little experiment in transformation.

Everyone, not just Carol, came to regard her hair as a symbol of things they cared about, as a way out of the sometimes stultifying Bodger traditions. What started out as a little liberating gesture for Carol ended up as a liberating gesture for the entire institution.

A Word About Grey

Traditionally, grey hair has been a sign of advancing age. People made a fuss about Barbara Bush's grey hair on the grounds that it made her look more like the President's mother than his wife. People are convinced that grey hair drains colour from the face. They say it bestows age upon us. In a world that has no rites of passage, we have come to treat grey hair as a notice from our hormones, as a reckoning on the body by the body that a new stage in life has begun.

Pat, a lawyer in her forties, told me she deliberately colours her hair grey

There is some notion here, a primitive one, that grey hair represents the ashes of youth. As youngsters, we have a profusion of hair. It all but gushes from our heads. The body is so blessed with health, so rich in its resources, so sheer in its vitality that it throws off hair in wild profusion. And gradually this begins to end. Hair begins to thin and grey, to coarsen. We suppose the furnaces of youth are slowing, that vitality is at an ebb.

We are also persuaded that grey hair is the beginning of the end of our individuality. People once distinguished by different colours all look the same. All those astonishingly various and vibrant blacks, browns, reds and blonds, all of them are turning into one single, monotonous grey.

But not everyone buys the idea that grey marks the beginning of the end of the expressive, vivid self. One of the women I interviewed, Pat, a lawyer in her forties, told me she deliberately colours her hair grey. She does it, she said, to give herself "*gravitas*," to give herself an air of wisdom and experience. "Hey, it works for men, right? Why shouldn't it for me?" And it does. Grey hair gives her beauty presence and tranquillity.

In 1993, grey became a passing fashion for English women in their twenties. A London department store reported that young women were using grey "as a fashion statement." Kathryn Hughes, the British journalist who spotted the trend, declared with some astonishment, "Suddenly it is cool to be grey."[20] Hughes talks about grey "highlights." When this term is applied to grey, you know things are starting to change.

But this is, for the moment, a minority opinion. Our culture has traditionally used grey as a pejorative term. "Grey" is what we call any featureless, oppressive world: prison, poverty, hospital, the Soviet Union. The days of November that threaten our good humour we call "grey."

Writing for *Redbook* magazine in 1991, Anna Qindlen reported a feeling of unease as grey hair appeared: "I don't look quite so much like myself anymore. I felt like I was beginning to fade."[21]

She would not mind, she said, going "good grey." But she was going "bad grey," "slowly and streakily." There is the fear of diminished sexual allure. There is a fear that things are ending. Colouring was not the answer. As Qindlen put it, "I somehow feel that coloring to cover gray belies the steady progression of life and the honorable nature of growing older."

What's really irritating is that grey is believed to make men more distinguished. As grey begins at the temples, the stereotype says, men are ready for high political or corporate office; the world should now look to them for sage advice and thoughtful counsel. We don't get much more sexist than this, do we? Women are made to pay for advancing age with their credibility and their attractiveness. Men are seen to be improved by it.

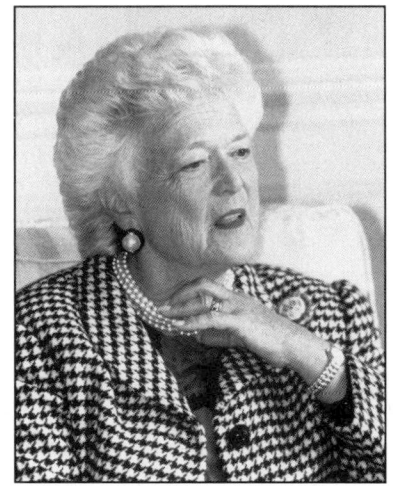

Barbara Bush: Controversial grey

There are women who do grey well. There's something about the way they go grey, and the way it suits their skin and eyes, that makes them striking. But not everyone is so blessed. For most of the world grey is, according to the stereotype, an aesthetic impairment, a blight upon one's looks.

Some women have set out to change all this. They now wear their grey as a badge of integrity and to embrace advancing age. They use it to insist that age holds no shame and induces no penalty. These women are pioneers in a heroic movement. They will pay a penalty until the penalty goes away. They will defy the "law" until it is rescinded.[22]

There are also honourable alternatives to grey. There is nothing wrong or mistaken about covering grey hair with another colour. Some women let their hair go grey because "I want to be the real me."[23] But it is worth remembering that in a transformational culture, there are many "real me"s. We are each of us the outcome of our self-constructive efforts. Our grey hair is no less the "real me" than the profuse hair we had as a teenager. It is simply the accident of our present biological condition, and no necessary marker of the authentic self.

Why give up transformational colours and bow to grey? To say that women *must* embrace grey is to bow to the stereotypes of age. It is to say that as they age people must give up their individuality. To insist on grey is to say, in effect, "Sorry, transformation is the liberty of youth and no one who values their dignity should do it in later years." This is, plainly, ageist nonsense.

For some women, the happy compromise is the use of colour to push back grey without eliminating it. Good colourists add just enough colour to prevent the overall impression of grey and whatever stigmatizing associations it carries, while enough is allowed to remain so that there is finally "truth in packaging."

We've come a long way since the days when a woman had to use the code word "treatments" to get her hair coloured. Those who now attack the covering of grey threaten to turn hair colouring back into a guilty secret. Let us not forsake this transformational liberty.

Make-overs of Style and Self:
Ten Options in the Current World of Hair

*T*here are a lot of hairstyles out there: parted-in-the-middle waif looks; towering, indomitable big hair; Shirley Temple ringlets; hair that is the very picture of boardroom professionalism; hair that is the very picture of bedroom sensuality; overpermed, Brillo-pad bad hair; hair that evokes Egypt; hair that is chicly European; hair that declares hippie abandon; hair that shouts status; hair that shouts stasis; hair that says "under construction, sorry for any inconvenience caused."

The many styles in the world of hair represent a map of many, if not most, of the possible selves in our culture. They are the envelope of possibilities every hairdresser consults when he or she sits down to establish a new look for a client. In the best-case scenario, each look is a new opportunity for the client's transformation and self-discovery. In the worst, each look is, aesthetically or emotionally, a dead end.

The bob and the blunt cut are essentially feminist inventions

These many styles have many meanings. "Voluptuous hair" is mostly about sexuality. "Imperial hair" is mostly about social standing. The "career coif" is mostly about professionalism. The "shaved and shorn" look is mostly about protest. The "Pixie" look is about a certain charm and élan. The "mature bob" is about a certain tragic or dignified retreat from fashion. Each look is a piece of our culture turned into the nature of hair.

These many styles have many origins. Some are from the world of haute coiffeur, some are from the teen world of 1950s California, while others are from ill-founded fantasies about forgotten empires and eras. And they come from a hundred different motives. The bob and the blunt cut are essentially feminist inventions. Imperial hair is the invention of an upper class. The shaved and shorn look was a punk invention, invented only thirty years ago in the streets of Manchester and London. And big hair was largely the work of the rural world of country and western. New styles can come to us from virtually anywhere.

The sheer number of styles out there reflects the new pluralism of the style world. In the early part of this century, every new fashion eclipsed every old fashion; it cleared the deck and wiped the slate clean. Not any more. Old fashions are no longer forced into obscurity; now they hang around even after new fashions emerge. So we live in a world that is filling up with options. We live on the edge of a great archaeological pool of possibilities. There are now upwards of forty or fifty identifiably different looks in the world of hair. We've got a lot to choose from.

Naturally, it was impossible to canvass all the looks out there. Instead, I chose ten to look at closely. Some got included because they were fashionable,

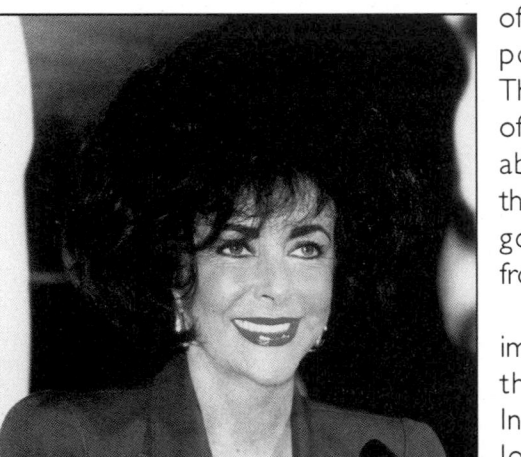

Liz Taylor: Big hair, the Hollywood version

some because they were popular, some because they were preposterous, some because they were curious, and some because they were just so damn big. They are not a perfect choice. They necessarily involve some overlap and some arbitrariness, they will allow us to consider a healthy cross-section of the contemporary world of hair.

Big Hair

- **The higher the hair, the nearer to God**
- **Guys who drive Camaros really like this**
- **You could take this off and put it on a shelf**

"Big hair" is one of the architectural marvels of our time. It stands high. It stands wide. It steps forward and demands to be seen. Big hair looks for impact, drama and extravagance. It's not much interested in cunning, subtlety, delicacy. And it doesn't care about natural. It's too busy defying gravity and getting our attention.

Big hair:
Love it or leave it

> I blow-dry it upside down, tease it out, gel it, mousse it and then spray the hell out of it.[1]

> I rat the tar out of it. I spray the hell out of it. We get it up there. We defy gravity.[2]

There is a lot of snobbery surrounding big hair. Some people in the world of fashion can't conceal their disdain. New Yorkers call it "bridge and tunnel:" that's their way of saying that nobody wears it inside the magic circle of Manhattan. Others say it's an "inland Florida" or "small-town" look. For some of the fashion world, this is a major "don't."

On the other hand, those who wear it defend it with a passion. Roger Thompson found this out when he opened a salon in a North Dallas mall. Thompson is a former artistic director for Vidal Sassoon in New York City, and his arrival in Dallas was awaited eagerly. But things went wrong from the beginning. To the astonishment of Dallas, Mr. Thompson refused, on point of principle, to do big hair. He was, after all, one of the generals in Sassoon's war against the bouffant.

Dallas was enraged. Local hairdressers accused Thompson's staff of being "snobs" and "twits." Dallas women called Thompson an élitist. "New Yorkers have such an attitude," one of them hissed. The implication was clear. Thompson could embrace local standards or he could take a hike. Big hair: love it or leave it.[3]

In fact, Thompson stayed on and now prospers in Dallas. He is one of several hairdressers in Dallas who give women alternatives to the big hair look. His salon is a kind of safe house for local women when they decide to give it up. But Thompson's "welcome" to Dallas gives us a glimpse of the intensity with which big hair supporters defend themselves against the disapproval of the main-stream hair community. It may be "bridge and tunnel" to some people, but it is high orthodoxy to those who wear it.

Women like big hair for many reasons. Some are aes-thetic: big hair makes even large and awkward facial fea-tures look delicate and petite. That hooter of a nose takes on a new proportion. Big ears disappear. Even command-ing chins recede. Big hair is also a lot cheaper than plastic surgery, and you don't need ten years of higher education to perform it.

Big hair is gregarious. This is Dolly Parton hair, and it helps in the construction of a Dolly Parton personality. This look is forthright. It has no pretensions and no airs. Big hair says, "What you see is what you get."

There is, incidentally, a second reason for big hair in the world of country and western: simple visibility. In order for a woman to have presence on the stage, she needs all the help she can get. As one hairdresser put it, "If you want anyone to see it past the tenth row, you got to pile it high."

Dolly Parton's hair gives women a place on the stage—in music and in life. It is the female equivalent of the ten gallon hat.

Big hair is also sexual. The women of Long Island are famous for very big hair. There isn't anything sexier, in their opinion, than hair that stands high and wide. One of them told me that she never knows which is worse, the smoke at the disco or the hairspray in the washroom. "You can't see for either one."

Long Island women claim big hair makes them look wild and outgoing. It's the outward promise of inward passion. The message is not lost on the men of Long Island. "It looks like something electric. They look aggressive, and I like aggressive girls."[4]

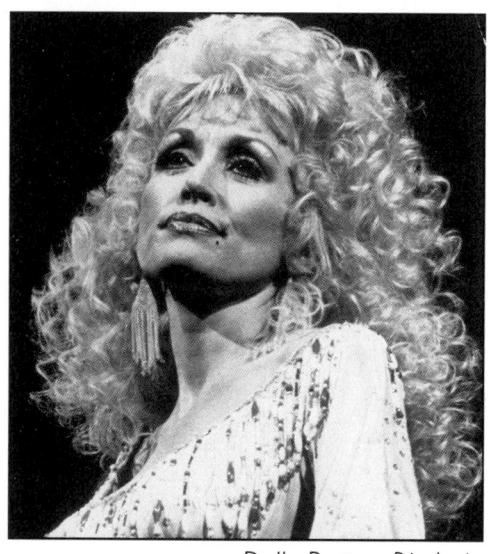

Dolly Parton: Big hair, the country and western version

And this raises a question. If the object is to look sexy, why not wear voluptuous hair in the sex-kitten style? Bighair wearers told me they regarded voluptuous hair as soft and weak. Not enough gumption, not enough gusto, they said. Big hair has the advantage of sending a come hither message, but it also creates a kind of armour: "You know who you're dealing with."

Big hair is loved by mall dolls. For them it says, 'I don't care about books, I care about guys." It is the simplest way for a mall doll to let the world know she is there to participate, not observe. Guys who like to drive Camaros apparently also like to have a mall doll with big hair beside them. Both the Camaro and the mall doll are status trophies.

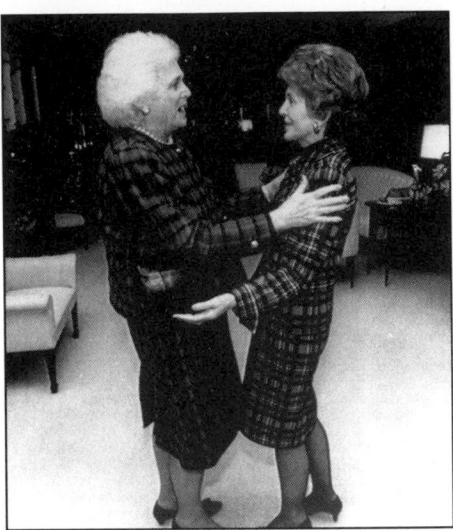

Barbara and Nancy:
Big hair, the White House version

Big hair has a certain authority. Under the right circumstances, it is a commanding look. The governor of Texas, Anne Richards, wears it extremely effectively. It's one of the most effective badges of office. Barbara Bush had a variation on big hair. So did Nancy Reagan. Elizabeth Taylor, the closest thing to royalty America has ever had, has been a champion of big hair for many years. The virtue of big hair is that it gives the wearer a certain size and majesty. It makes her imposing.

Big hair says, "Take me seriously, I do." It is a statement of self-regard. This is not a feminist cut, but it has, among other things, a variation on the feminist message: "Do not trifle with me, bucko." This is how it is worn by the formidable Julia Sugarbaker character on TV's "Designing Women."

The enemies of big hair say a lot of nasty things. They say it makes a woman look cheap and vulgar. They say it is worn by older women to look younger and by younger women to look older. They say women use it as a substitute for confidence. They say women wear it for the same reason that men drive powerful cars, to compensate for feelings of inadequacy. They say women use big hair to hide behind. They say that big hair is a downward cycle of teasing and damage, until big hair becomes a necessity instead of a choice. They say this is the most unsensual look in the world: men can't run their hands through it. And the final dig: big hair is anti-ecological; it demands lots and lots of hairspray.

Poof and Woof Hair: Little Big Hair

"Poof and woof" hair is an important variation on big hair. It happens when women add body and shape to their hair by teasing the bangs and/or the crown and/or the hair around the face.

Girls in high school use spot-teasing once they get to school. And then they undo it before they go home. Mom never has to know. This is big hair on tap.

Poof and woof hair has a purpose, teenagers told me: "You poof your hair and the guys go woof. Poof and woof. That's what my friend says."

Teenage boys are not the world's most gifted semioticians, but we can assume that the semaphore of the spot-tease does get through to them. (Whether they actually woof in response is perhaps less certain. As your humble ethnographer, I have no confirmed sighting of the woof response. I did not see or hear one for myself.)

Spot-teasing is extremely popular at some malls these days. But it is not only teenage girls who consider it the style of choice. Women of all ages wear it with enthusiasm. The best spot-teasing is great architecture. It adds form, drama and presence to the wearer. It frames the face. And when the wearer is a blonde, it frames the face with light.

The trouble is that sometimes the wearer thinks only about the face. We've all seen it: a woman who looks elaborately coiffed from the front but neglected from the sides and back. (The best example is a woman with naturally bone-straight hair who uses a curling iron and teasing on

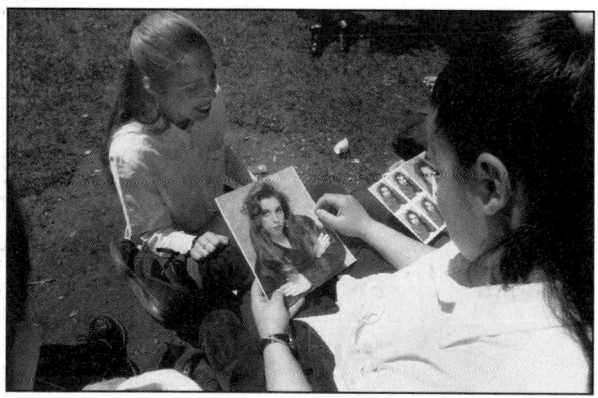

Teen contemplates poof and woof options

her bangs.) Hairdressers describe this with despair. Clients will give them very explicit instructions about the hair around the face. And when the hairdresser asks, "Well, what about the back?" the answer is often, "Oh, I don't know, do what you want, I never see the back."

The enemies of poof and woof and other instances of spot-teasing are legion. One woman told me: "Their priority is the way they look. It's shallow. It doesn't look natural. It doesn't look like it grew out of anybody's head.

Big hair of this kind is probably indestructible. It is despised by the world of fashion. It was attacked by the Sassoon revolution. It was ridiculed during the hippie revolution of the 1960s. It is routinely belittled by hairdressers. Worn by teenagers, it has endured the contempt of parents, school officials, high fashion, polite society and just about everyone else. And it has survived it all. This is one hardy haircut.

The Historical Note

Big hair is, of course, not the exclusive domain of women. Englishmen in the 1770s wore their hair so big they made a spectacle of themselves. They were called Macaronis (after their favourite Italian dish) and they wore "furiously powdered" wigs that towered over their heads. In order to exaggerate the size of these wigs, Macaronis wore very small hats.[5]

By the 1780s women's hair, too, had reached into the heavens, ornamented by an assortment of things: plumes, flowers, fruit, ribbons, lace and bits of blown glass, sometimes all at once. They appeared in public with miniature gardens or naval engagements played out in their hair.[6] The hair of the period grew so large that really thoughtful hosts rebuilt doorways so that guests could enter the room without destroying the little theatres on their heads.

It seems unlikely that the women who wore these vast hairdos were doing so on their own behalf. Almost certainly they were engaging in what American economist

Thorstein Veblen called "surrogate consumption:" they were demonstrating not their own but their husbands' status and wealth.[7]

Here is a description of one woman's hairdo in England around 1794:

> A chiffonet of Italian gauze, the bandeau composed of 3 rows of white pearls, 2 rows of the same pearls twisted round the chiffonet. 3 plain white feathers and 2 edged with lilac placed in the head-dress. Bell lapets of gauze, tied in different parts with pearls. The hair very lightly frizzed, thrown into a variety of curls and ringlets and intermixed with the chiffonet.[8]

Men and women were wearing hairdos with all the complexity of a planetary system.

Big hair slipped from fashion as a result of the republican styles that prevailed after the French Revolution. And we see it appear and disappear, comet-like, over the next two hundred years. It has put in several spectacular appearances in our own century. It appeared at the turn of the century, only to be challenged, as we shall see, by the bob. It appeared once more in the 1950s as the staple of the old world of hair in North America.

In the 1960s it ran through the teen world, in the words of the *New York Times*, like a "tidal wave."[9] Teens wore the "chemise," in which the hair took the shape of a bubble with two cheek curls, the "beehive,"

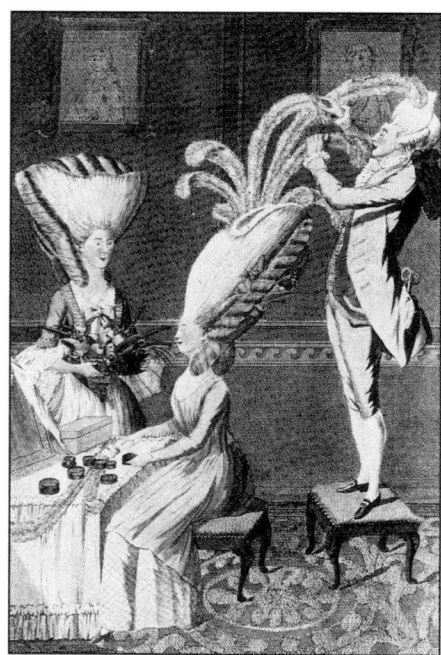

Big hair of history:
18th-century women's hair

a cone that rose from the head, and the "flip," a high puff-ball above that turned up at the ends. Annette Funicello, Sandra Dee, Mary Tyler Moore and Doris Day all wore the flip. This look was joined by "frou frou" curls, these worn on the smooth surface of teased hair.[10] (They may be the immediate ancestor of spot-teasing.)

> *Where big hair lives, it thrives. And where it prevails, it is indomitable.*

The "guiche" was another device of the bouffant period.[11] This was a curl that appeared on both cheeks. The guiche could be worn with any other style, including the chemise, but it needed the height of well-teased hair to work at all. The trouble with the guiche-bouffant combination was that it was so large and daunting that it gave some women a water buffalo look.

> With several variations in the hairdo, one thing is constant: a high, puffed-up effect that is achieved by painstaking teasing. This is a process in which each lock is combed backward until the hair stands straight up. Then it is carefully patted into place without losing any of the height.[12]

Big hair returned periodically and fitfully in the 1970s and 1980s. A rock group from Georgia, the B-52s, revived it, as did the late-night TV cult figure Elmira. Neither created a mainstream trend.

On the whole, big hair has almost never been welcome in the mainstream. But it has lived on in Texas, in the South, on Long Island, in the world of country and western music and, among teenagers, in suburban malls. The *Wall Street Journal* recently announced the "decline" of big hair and the onset of "dark days for lacquered dos."[13] But the press is always reporting the death of big hair. It's just wishful thinking. Where big hair lives, it thrives. And where it prevails, it is indomitable.

The Minority Opinion

Guys who drive Camaros *do* like this look. So do guys who live on Long Island and men with an affinity for country and western. Men of the heartland of North America have always liked this look. Some of them plainly like big hair now for the same reason men liked it in the 1950s: because it feels like an act of deference by women to men. It is women radically transforming themselves in order to make themselves attractive (in the manner of high heels and push-up bras). But other men see this look as many women intend them to: as a statement of self-regard and gusto. They told me, in effect, they like women who like themselves. Big hair says this loud and clear.

Some other men regard big hair as old-fashioned and unattractive. One just laughed when I showed him a picture. "There are still women like this?" he exclaimed. For some men this is the opposite of voluptuous hair. "I don't even want to touch it."

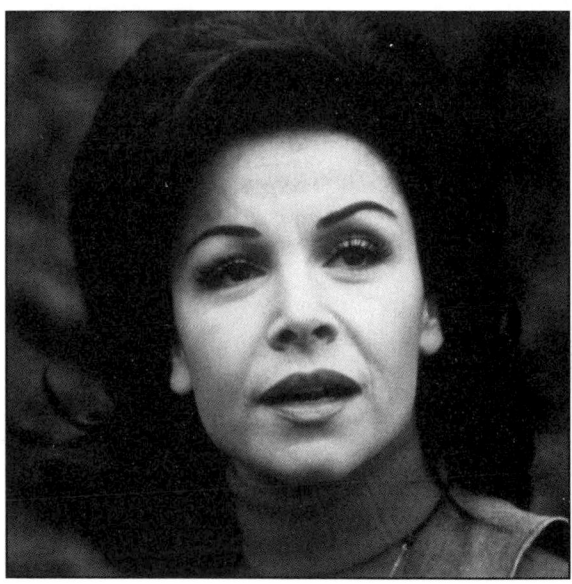

Annette Funicello: Classic flip

Voluptuous Hair

- **Wild and free**
- **This is the kind of a cut that gets a girl in trouble**
- **This is *vavoom* hair, this is "just had sex" hair**

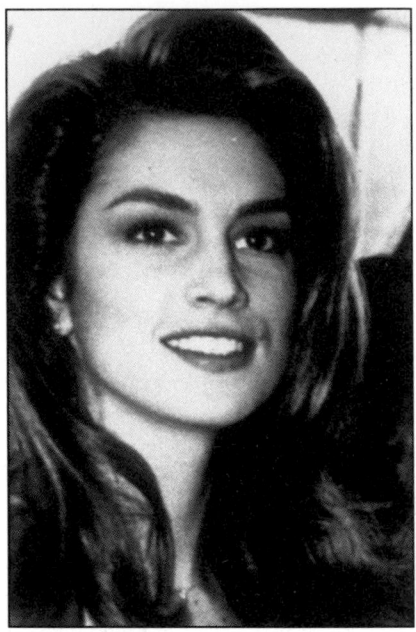

Cindy Crawford: Voluptuous hair

"Voluptuous hair" is "statement hair." The first thing it says is "youth." For a moment, all the women on "Beverly Hills 90210" (with one exception) had long hair, and they wore it as a statement of their eligibility.[14] This is a look many women wear in their teens and in their twenties. You can get away with it in your thirties, but the clock is ticking. (Cindy Crawford is still wearing it, for instance.) For many women, long hair is one of the liberties of youth.

Second, voluptuous hair has a sexual message. As Christophe of Beverly Hills puts it, "Sexy hair is long, in the eyes. That just-out-of-bed thing." John Sahag says the same. "Sexy means that throwaway look, never too set and controlled."[15] Long hair says the wearer is a sexual creature.

The sexual message comes easily to voluptuous hair. Long hair is, after all, abundant hair. When correctly styled, it has the appearance of being wild and uncontained. Hair and sex, in our culture, have been given this wildness in common.

Long hair is also associated with sex because of its sensual texture. As writer Claire Scovell puts it, "Men love to weave their fingers into *Voluptuous hair* a heavy skein of thick hair, and there's noth-*makes for* ing more sensual than the brush of lengthy *voluptuous bodies* locks upon a naked chest—his or yours."[16] Also, long hair holds perfume well, and this contributes something to the abandon of the moment. So speak some men.

Hollywood has made an important contribution to all of this. One of the movie's stock images is the transformation that takes place when a woman (typically a librarian) removes her glasses, unbuttons her blouse, and, most important, lets down her hair. The television series "Cheers" used the convention to transform Lilith from ice princess into temptress. The external transformation is supposed to suggest an internal one: a woman moving from a nervous bureaucratic mode to something wild, free and profusely sexual. Thus has Hollywood helped to identify the sexual significance of voluptuous hair.

And advertising has made its contribution as well. A recent Revlon ad shows Cindy Crawford and Claudia Schiffer together. The headline reads "Outrageous Body! Outrageous Shine." Crawford and Schiffer are wearing their signature looks: long, full hair that can only be described as voluptuous. The ad turns on a familiar, if unconscious, pun: hair with great body endows bodies with great body. Voluptuous hair makes for voluptuous bodies. In this case, the fullness and the curves of the hair are symbolically conso-

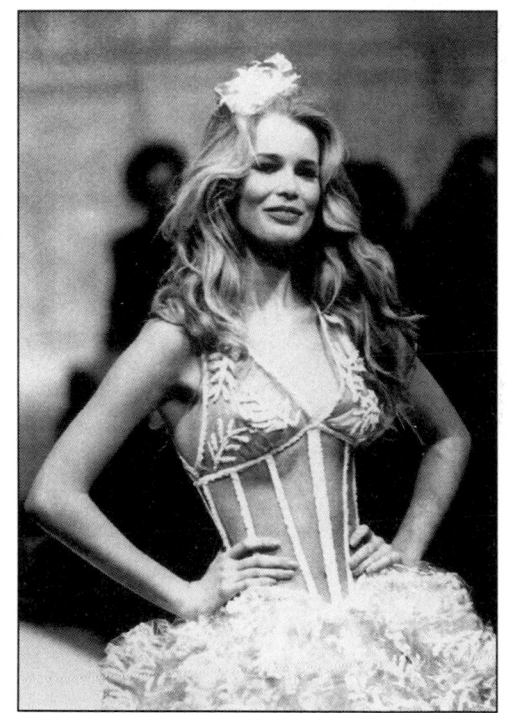

Claudia Schiffer: More voluptuous hair

nant with the fullness and the curves of the body below.

The fashion magazines have made a contribution of their own. Here is *Harper's Bazaar* extolling the virtues of long hair.

…one thing is guaranteed to make a man stop and stare with unadulterated delight—long, lustrous hair. For many, the mere sight can arouse desire to reach out and caress it; crowded elevators can be a constant test of self-control.[17]

If it's beginning to seem that the link between long hair and sexuality is just an invention of Hollywood and the fashion world, bear in mind that this conviction is embedded in the very stuff of American popular culture. Take, for instance, the way hair figures in the graduation prom. For the first part of the evening, and the official part of the rite of passage, hair is worn up. The teen is stepping into adulthood, and the more formal she looks, the more ready she is for the transition. And then the second, unofficial part of the prom takes place. Teens let their hair down and give themselves over to abandon. Long, wild hair stands for their new sexual licence and other adult freedoms. Again, long hair represents the transition into sexuality.

"flipping" was first officially identified by two social scientists in 1989

Long hair is not just about sex; it's also about romance. Long hair is a symbol of a state of emotional exaltation, in which sensitivities and sensibilities have been heightened by romantic engagement. It is virtually impossible for us to imagine a romantic heroine with short hair. Here's how a college student put it:

> I'm always a true romantic at heart, which is why I think I've always wanted my hair long. I've always associated long, beautiful hair with romance, just like the heroines in the Harlequin Romance novels I read when I was younger.[18]

Paradoxically, long hair can also sometimes have an *Alice in Wonderland* look to it, and in this case it is the opposite of sexual. It declares the innocence of childhood and a time when there is no sexual motive or knowledge. The childlike waif-type version of long hair has the same childlike non-sexual character as the *Alice in Wonderland* cut.

The '90s have also seen a revival of the hippie cut, in which hair is worn long, parted in the middle and feathered at the tips. This was the look Kate Moss brought to her meteoric rise in the fashion world: waifish, boyish, distracted and otherworldly.[19] This look has a romantic quality, except when worn in a grunge manner. In this case, it's a declaration of radical naturalism. It's about sex,

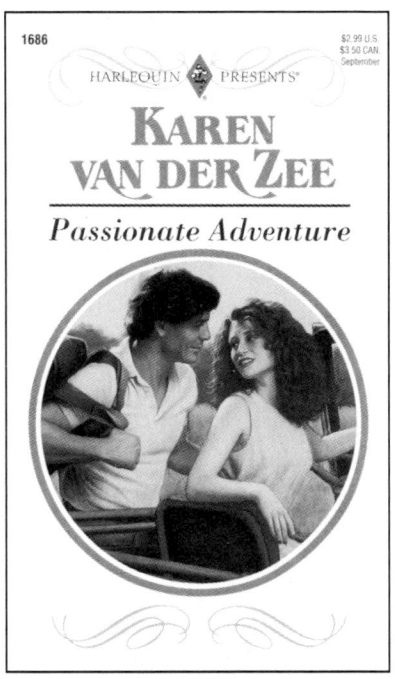

but it's also about everything else untrammelled by civilization and its discontents.

Women with long hair tend to touch and flip it. In fact, the practice of "flipping" was first officially identified by two social scientists, Monica Moore and Diana Butler, in 1989. Moore and Butler watched the ways teenage girls smile, scan the room, lick their lips, head toss and "hair flip." Unfortunately, Moore and Butler give no formal account of flipping.[20] We must fashion our own account of this crucial use of voluptuous hair.

There was something fascinating about the way her appearance changed almost continually as the lunch wore on

One of the things the flip says is, "Pay attention." In fact, in our sexist culture, this is one of the few ways that a teenage girl can attract the attention of a boy—anything more obvious is off limits. This is the way it works in the movie *About Last Night ...*, with Rob

Lowe and Demi Moore. Moore's character watches newly acquainted male and female characters interacting at a bar. Even at a distance, she can see the relationship maturingly nicely. "Here comes the flip," she says, just seconds before the female produces it.

The nice thing about the hair flip is that it's easy to repudiate. If the guy gets the message and makes his approach, and you decide you've made a mistake, it's easy enough to send him packing. After all, you didn't actually issue a formal invitation. And if the little jerk fails to respond, well, you can pretend you never sent him a signal in the first place. ("God! I was just adjusting my hair!") Hair flipping is, to this extent, a relatively risk-free way of sending a message.

But flipping is also used for another purpose. Early in the research for this book, I happened to have lunch with a woman in Toronto. As lunch progressed I couldn't help but notice that she was almost constantly rearranging her hair, moving it from one side of her head to the other, variously shaping and reshaping it.

It would be easy to flatter myself and imagine she was sending me a message about her interest in me, but it would be wrong. In fact, I think she was constantly shifting her image, to say, in effect, "Don't make any glib assumptions, I am never the same woman: I transform myself before your very eyes." And it worked. There was something fascinating about the way her appearance changed almost continually as the lunch wore on. And all of this communicated itself on an unconscious level.

I have since talked to women about this kind of hair flipping and most of them just laugh. They treat it as a gesture of vanity, as one of the things of childhood that you must put behind you. One of them said, "Oh God, that's the old thing, isn't it? A woman changing her appearance to hold a man's attention. Those days have passed. Hair flipping has gone the way of high-heeled shoes—men may like them, but we've had enough."

There is a third reason, however, for hair touching and flipping. Picture the gangster's moll in a '40s movie. She spends much of her time patting her hair in a bored, thoughtless way that says, "I have several hundred better uses for my time." When I see this gesture in the movies, or its latter-day equivalent at the mall, I can't help wondering whether it doesn't say, "I take myself very seriously. If you have any thoughts of approaching, you'd better do the same." This version of the flip or the pat is a measure of self-regard.

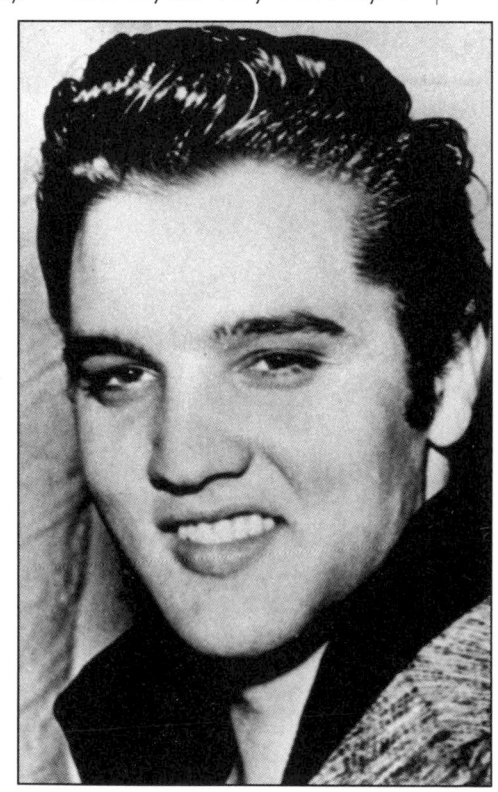

It's worth pointing out that hair flipping and touching is not restricted to women. Elvis made a positive fetish of touching his hair. In his stage performance he was constantly drawing his hand back across well-greased hair. This became a kind of signature gesture for the '50s male (and the Fonz in the '50s TV revival "Happy Days"). The gesture was about self-regard and sexual charisma. We don't see it much these days. Generally, men are supposed to leave their hair alone.

The Historical Note

Long hair as a sign of youth, vitality and sexuality is everywhere in the western tradition. In the classical world, long hair was frequently used as a sign of disordered emotions, of the passions on a rampage. When the Greek dramatist

Euripides has women give themselves over to sexual abandon in *The Bacchae*, he shows them on the hillside, their "hair streaming behind."[21]

In seventeenth-century Europe, the Englishman John Aubrey observed:

> At Leghorn, and other Ports in Italie, when Shippes arrive, the Courtizans runne to the Mariners with their Lutes and Ghitarres, playing and singing, with their Haire dissheveld, and Breasts naked, to allure them.[22]

The Victorians built a cult around hair, and they too equated hair and sexual character.

> … the more abundant the hair, the more potent the sexual invitation it implied.[23]

The bob helped to discourage big hair in the twentieth century, and it wasn't until the war years that it made a real comeback. In 1941, Veronica Lake appeared in *I Wanted Wings* with long, shoulder-length locks. The nation went wild. *Life* magazine was breathless with enthusiasm, declaring hers the most influential haircut since Jean Harlow's in the 1930s. Lake's hair was now as famous, *Life* claimed, as Fred Astaire's feet or Dietrich's legs.[24]

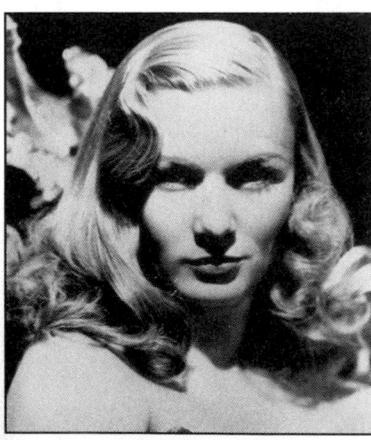

Veronica Lake: The most influential hair since Harlow

But this was just the beginning. The connection between long hair and sex was not yet fully fashioned. Long hair was not yet voluptuous. In the 1950s, long hair had to fight it out with the big hair bouffants of the period. Besides, the great sex stars were not wearing it. Marilyn Monroe did not adopt it. Nor did her great contemporary, Jayne Mansfield. America's sexuality continued to keep its hair relatively short.

Once more, a critical influence came from abroad. Brigitte Bardot established the definitive "sex-kitten" role in Roger Vadim's 1957 film ... *And God Created Woman.* Long hair and sexual charisma were now linked. The new sex-kittens were about to make long hair voluptuous hair.

Suddenly, women like Jackie Onassis, then Mrs. John F. Kennedy, were taking their cue from college girls

By 1966, when Raquel Welch appeared in *One Million Years B.C.*, the choice was clear. In order to turn Welch into a jungle tigress, the studio resorted to animal skins and voluptuous hair. The tradition burgeoned. Ursula Andress and Claudia Cardinale perpetuated and refined the sex-kit-

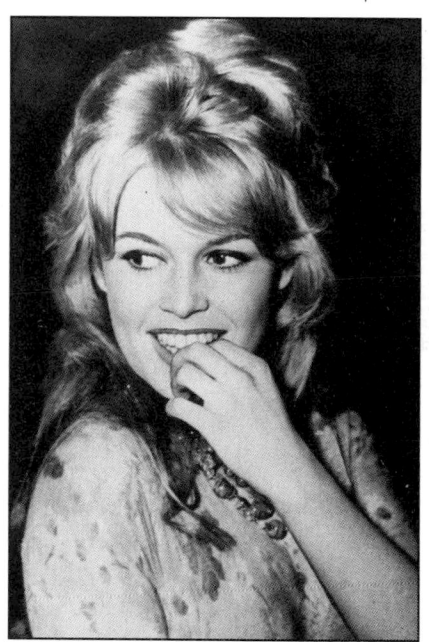

ten tradition. Andress was one of several stars to start her career in the James Bond movies. The Bond women were nothing if not sexual, and by this time it was simply inevitable that all of them have voluptuous hair.

The 1960s saw the rise of yet another competitor: ironed hair. Young women were taking long hair and ironing it absolutely flat.[25] This removed voluptuous curls and sensual movement. The new look created a sensation. Millions of teenage and college women with naturally curly hair spent part of

Brigitte Bardot: Sex-kitten hair

each morning with their hair on the ironing board.

To everyone's astonishment, this invention of the new and strange youth culture was beginning to have an influence on the rest of society. The ironed look trickled up to influence mature women and polite society. Suddenly, women like Jackie Onassis, then Mrs. John F. Kennedy, were taking their cue from college girls. *The New York Times* declared: "Hairdressers predict that the elaborate cushioned hairdos and cascading pigtails of gala evenings will soon be replaced by long straight hair that is swept behind the ears and falls down, down, down."[26]

The '70s saw a return of voluptuous hair. The stars of the day included Christie Brinkley, Lindsay Wagner and Farrah Fawcett. "Charlie's Angels" became the TV equivalent of the Bond series, launching the careers of several women with long hair and a sexual charisma. And this time the competitors were fewer and less powerful. Now virtually everyone under twenty-one had a poster of one of the new sex-kittens in his or her bedroom. Voluptuous hair was everywhere.

> *Increasingly, voluptuous hair said "bimbo"*

But the sex-kitten convention had returned only to calcify into a terrible cliché. Voluptuous hair began to stand for two things: sexuality and not much acting ability. Increasingly, it said "bimbo." Hollywood had succeeded in turning yet another of its conventions into self-parody. The Sassoon revolution was well underway. Feminism was on the rise. Voluptuous hair was increasingly important for young women. It was the cut of choice for the mall. But it was losing fans downtown and in professional circles.

In the 1980s, the tradition was perpetuated by the likes of Kim Basinger and Daryl Hannah. (Basinger was another graduate of the James Bond sex-kitten academy.) Now, in the '90s voluptuous hair is worn by the likes of Cindy Crawford and Claudia Schiffer. In 1991 it was recommended by that god of the hairdressing world Oribe, who has created voluptuous hairstyles for several of his clientele. He has also publicly called for a look that is "deliberately dishevelled."[27]

Recently, voluptuous hair found a strange and unexpected partner. The rise of "biker chic," which itself sounds like a contradiction in terms, has encouraged some women to wear hair that is long and tousled. This is another "trickle up" fashion influence, and an unlikely one. *Rolling Stone* magazine has called the look something between "menacing and seductive." New York City hairstylist Thom Priano is quoted as saying, "I've never believed in neat hair. People always touch their hair. Hair has to look real for it to be sexy."[28]

The Minority Opinion

Men understand voluptuous hair. They believe it's for them. It has volume, movement, length and mass. It is sensual and inviting. It plays out the properties of sex itself; it is wild and unconstrained. They see it as a promise of sensuality.

This is the look men respond to with the greatest force and clarity, and this makes it a great selection device. Women who want the enthusiastic and sexual attentions of men know exactly what to wear. Women who wish to avoid these attentions know exactly what to avoid. You can "edit out" a great deal of unwanted male attention by steering clear of this kind of hair.

No one has yet attempted to rehabilitate this look: it remains a way of soliciting traditional male attention, for better and for worse. There is one candidate for the job, however. Feminist author Naomi Wolf wears this cut. She resists every sexist stereotype. She expresses dismay at the manner in which women are treated like objects in our society. But she also wears the single most sexual and stereotyped haircut in the stylistic envelope. This is puzzling. Either Ms. Wolf is not paying attention to the cultural significance of her haircut, or she means to transform its significance.

Imperial Hair

- This cut makes you listen to what she says
- Don't rub this one the wrong way, she might bite

• **This is high society, this is someone with power**

"Imperial hair" is big hair with a purpose. This is hair with political clout. It says "I am a woman to be reckoned with." This is the haircut favoured by women like former British prime minister Margaret Thatcher and Kathleen Graham, editor of the *Washington Post*. It works best when women have power and don't care, and don't have to care, who will take offence.

> ### *Imperial hair is big hair with a purpose*

This cut positions itself skilfully. There is nothing "wild and free" about it. It is attractive but it is not particularly sexual or inviting. It dispenses with the very notion that the wearer is someone who welcomes or depends upon sexual attention from men. This cut doesn't need to be winning: it has already won.

Imperial hair is relatively immobile, the antithesis of the feathered, wispy or trailing look. There is nothing emotionally expressive or accommodating about it. This cut says, "I know exactly what I want. And I am not prepared to change. Not for you, at any rate." This haircut is decisive and emphatic. It holds out no promise of compromise or negotiation. Though not exactly vain, it is supremely self-confident. It says that the wearer believes in herself without a shadow of a doubt: "I know exactly who I am. I may or may not be interested in who you are."

This cut is useful for a professional woman in the later years of her career. It is

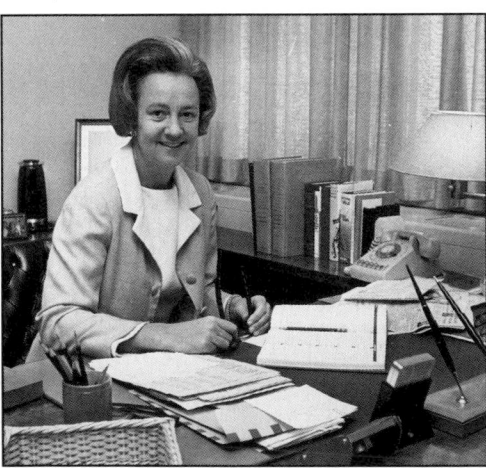

Kathleen Graham: Uncompromising hair

precisely wrong for a professional woman in the early years of her career, and probably just too matronly for any younger woman, period. It is too inflexible, too closed, too self-assured, too self-important to look good on anyone who is just creating an identity for herself. But for the established professional or socialite, this cut is a formidable show of strength.

You can see why this cut served Margaret Thatcher so well. It let people know that the Iron Lady was resolute and, in her famous phrase, "not for turning."

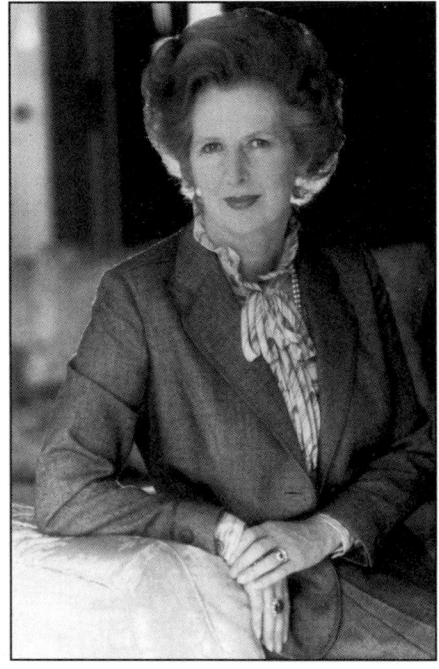

Margaret Thatcher: Hair as Nation

Interestingly, Mrs. Thatcher began with an extremely rigid cut, a kind of "hair as helmet" effect, and moved later to a cut that was somewhat softer.[29] But even the later cuts had a trademark rigidity.

Mrs. Thatcher's hair was a perfect model of her nation. It was profuse and celebrated the abundance Tory policy promised 1980s England. (Ronald Reagan's profuse hair had this same significance for 1980s America.) And it was coherent, the very picture of a nation bending itself to a single will.

Women rulers have long faced the particular challenges of sexism, in which some part of the nation harbours grave misgivings about a woman's ability to manage affairs of state. Elizabeth I responded to this challenge by cultivating the elaborate and splendid symbolism of her court. Were she alive today, she would certainly have used this cut to tell the world she was indomitable.

The down-sides of this cut are several. First, it is threatening to anyone who is uncomfortable with a woman wielding power. Second, it is sometimes seen to be rigid and controlling. In this case, the rigidness of the cut is seen to be an indication of a rigidness of management style and personality. Third, some women have said that the woman who wears this kind of cut "is not her own woman; she is controlled by someone." The alternative reading was, "This woman is using someone else's power." I don't know where this comes from, and the respondents were unable to tell me. It may be a residue of the sexist idea that a woman's power must be borrowed from some male source, that it cannot be her own.

The Minority Opinion

Predictably, men find this look a little daunting. They also find it highly readable. This look sends them a clear message on all frequencies. In terms of age, it says, "I am mature." In terms of status, it says, "I am upper middle class." In terms of gender, it says, "I am forthright, capable and not at all girlish." In terms of personality, it says, "I am confident."

The Murphy Brown Mane

- Hey, it's the late '70s!
- Hey, it's Murphy Brown!
- Hey, hold the hairspray!

This look manages to combine sex, sweetness and authority and makes them work together

This look is much loved by many of the women I talked to. Certainly, some people declared it old-fashioned and out of touch, but those who liked it absolutely loved it.

The secret of the look is that it combines sex, sweetness and authority, and if the history of hair tells us anything, it tells us that these three things almost never go together. Sex usually costs you authority. Sweetness usually costs you sex. Authority usually costs you sweetness. This look manages to combine sex, sweetness and authority, and makes them work together.

This look was largely crafted by two people, Farrah Fawcett and Candice Bergen as Murphy Brown. Between them, Fawcett and Bergen/Brown invented something remarkable.

Fawcett came to prominence in 1977, a star in the series of the moment, "Charlie's Angels," and wife of the male of the moment, Lee Majors. She was immediately influential. "I think she's the worst actress in the world," said a New York fan, "but I love her hair."[30] Millions of women and men felt the same way. Fawcett's influence was increased by her poster, which sold some three million copies.[31]

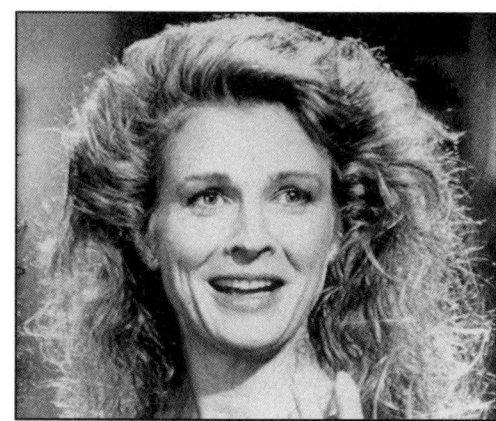

Candice Bergen: The Murphy Brown mane

One of the things that brought Fawcett to stardom was her hair. This was the creation of either Allen Edwards, Hugh York or Fawcett herself, depending on who you talk to. It was a layered cut, frosted and enlarged until it captured the very essence of California. Fawcett wanted it to look "free, wild and above all natural."[32] She created a look that captured the fitness, exuberance and energy of California. Fawcett managed to tap into that good-natured voltage for which the American female, especially the West Coast version thereof, has long been famous.

Fawcett has been accused of being a "Barbie Doll" beauty[33] but this misses the point. Fawcett's hair was powerful because it managed to capture California's cult of the body. It stood for health, vigour, vitality and the sensuality of perfect fitness.

Every interview done with Fawcett in the late 1970s details with devoted interest her workout regime, and she talks endlessly of her commitment to body. Notions of femaleness were under reconstruction here, including that most important symbol, the "woman's glow." For Fawcett this was simple. "I think every woman looks great after a good sweat."[34]

> *It's as if Fawcett's cut grew up and made it in the real world*

The strategy is consistent with the "unthreatening sexuality" Marilyn Monroe managed to create. Fawcett is sexual, but there is nothing steamy, exaggerated, pouting or crude about her appeal. This is "girl next door" winningness.

Fawcett had found another way to make sex available but unthreatening. Yes, she was braless, but that famous poster pose reassured us that she was also completely unmysterious, agreeable, open and forthcoming. Sex without the stigma. Here was a woman steamy enough for a young man to want on his wall. Here was a woman of sufficient innocence that his parents didn't mind.

We know where this cut's sex and sweetness come from. Fawcett managed to yoke them together in that great American tradition established by Monroe. But what about the authority of the look? How did this become a power look?

Enter Candice Bergen. On the head of FYI journalist Murphy Brown, this look has broadened its horizons and filled out its expressive potential. In fact, Candice Bergen has been good to and for the look. She has maintained its cheerful sexuality and added something new. And she has given it a resourcefulness it did not have before. Now the look is taking on that "devil-may-care, shoot from the hip, take or leave it" insouciance that Bergen does so well as Murphy Brown.

Murphy Brown is inexorable. She says what she wants, gets what she wants and goes where she wants. She is a perfect blonde in all of this. There is nothing complicated, mysterious or ineffable about her. What you see is exactly what you get. But no longer is the blondness a gesture of deference. There is no passivity, reticence or delicacy here. Not a trace.

It's as if Fawcett's cut grew up and made it in the real world. This is a cut with purpose, intensity and will. Like all good blond hair, it declares itself a long way off, but unlike most blond hair, it never lets up. This version of big hair keeps coming at you. The good thing about this authority look is that it is relatively unthreatening, both to men and to women. I can't help but think that this is the populist appeal of the Fawcett look speaking through.

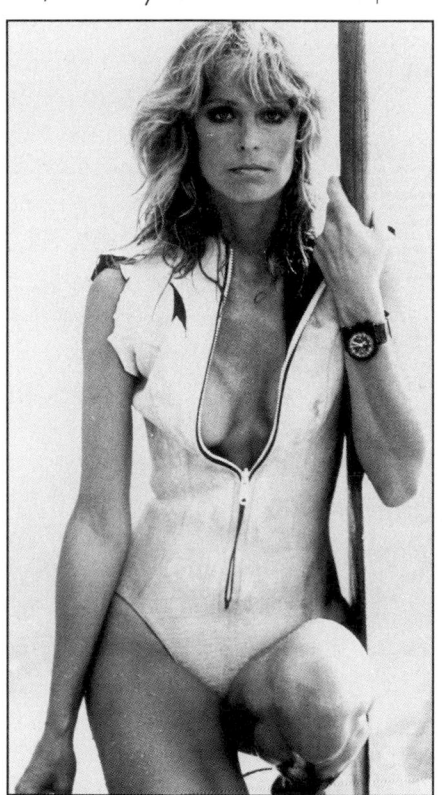

Farrah Fawcett: The California mane

However, the look is not without its weaknesses. First, this look is now the mall doll's idea of glamour. You cannot visit a North American suburb without seeing a great many of these haircuts, often accomplished with bleach and a reckless curling iron. This look does not stand up well to bad imitation, and in the wrong hands it turns quickly into self-parody.

Second, the look is seen by some younger women to be old-fashioned: too much hairspray, too much effort, not enough naturalism. "This is stuffed hair," said one. The wildness message of this hair depends on hair that can move. When it is frozen into place with hairspray, people are unhappy. The look has contradicted itself.

Third, the influence of Murphy Brown over this cut is now so powerful that the people who do not like her often do not like the cut. Fourth, some people see this as a mature woman's attempt to look young. "Mutton dressed as lamb," was the way one person put it.

Fifth, feminists often hate this cut and identify it as a capitulation to everything men demand: length, volume and "sexiness." Sixth, non-feminists often see it exactly the other way around. For them, this cut is bossy, self-important and insufficiently feminine. Seventh, some people see this as a middle-class person putting on airs, as the cut of someone who is trying to look upper class. They complain the cut has no subtlety.

The Minority Opinion

Men like this cut on the whole. It signals self-confidence and a certain friendliness. It promises a certain lack of guile, a certain straightforwardness. This is a good haircut for a woman to have when she has several male subordinates. It is feminine and sexual but it is also forthcoming. Men get the authority message quite clearly.

All men understand it, but not all of them like it. One or two said that this cut says the wearer "is not very flexible." One of them said this is an "I know best" haircut, as if the cut were somehow a symbol for bossiness. Sometimes the "authority" message speaks too loudly. But then, for some men, *any* authority message from a woman speaks too loudly.

The Pixie

- Feminine without being fussy
- Pixie, what a name! What's it from, the Brownies?

This cut has everything going for it. It's winning, versatile, fashionable and interesting. Most important, it has no enemies. And we can't say this of any other haircut.

The "Pixie" cut has no trade-offs. Women say it's fashionable without being risky, high-profile but low-maintenance, feminine but not old-fashioned. They like the look because it is unassuming and unshowy. There is, they say, nothing self-dramatizing about it. Finally, the Pixie cut is attractive without being overtly

> *This look has no snobbery, no competitive edge, no self-importance and no big sexual message*

sexual. It lets a woman declare her sexuality without provoking the "woof" response that sometimes greets long blond hair.

The Pixie is a companionable look. It says a woman has made an effort, that she wants to look attractive, but it also says that she is not trying to steal anyone's thunder (or her mate). The Pixie cut doesn't try to turn every head or stop every car. People like its unassuming quality. This look has no snobbery, no competitive edge, no self-importance and no big sexual message. It is perfectly balanced: attractive but not threatening.

There are four variations of the Pixie cut. One is the "super chic" variation. This variation is shorter and sharper than the everyday Pixie. In this guise, the cut starts to take on a certain elegance and hauteur. This is the Pixie as you see it on fashionable European women. This Pixie cut is a great statement of self-regard. It says, "My beauty is mostly for me. If you like it, fine. If you do not like it, that's fine, too. I do it for myself." This is the most assuming version of the cut.

Four women helped to introduce this chic, European variation to America. They were Audrey Hepburn and Leslie Caron at the beginning of the 1950s, and Françoise Sagan and Jean Seberg towards the end of the decade. Among them, they gave the look new credentials. They made it a refuge for women who wished to escape the big hair enthusiasms of 1950s America and embrace something more continental, artistic, sophisticated and even slightly *demi-monde*. The Pixie was a way out of the '50s construction of self.

The second variation is the "sassy" Pixie. It is playful, saucy, impudent and irreverent. The sassy Pixie has to be worn correctly, with a certain verve and panache—not everyone can pull it off. For the right woman, it is a great statement. The woman who wears the sassy Pixie can challenge conventional opinion. She can banter, bandy, cut and thrust. She can transcend "niceness" and get to grips with the world. And she can do all of this without making people run screaming from the room. The sassy Pixie is provocative but not antagonistic, playful, not aggressive. It tells people to be on guard but reassures them that they needn't take offence. It gives a woman some room in the world. The best example of this version of the Pixie is worn by Liza Minnelli, a long-time champion of the look and its persona.

The third variation is the "waif" Pixie. It makes a woman appear childlike and a little lost. In fact, in the 1950s this cut was actually sometimes called "the motherless child."[35] The champion of this look was Audrey Hepburn, who in 1954 "launched an altogether new type of beauty: a wistful waif, large-eyed, short-haired, minus all aids to beauty."[36] (Hepburn managed to contribute to both the super chic and the waif versions of the Pixie.) This Pixie is the look of the ingenue.

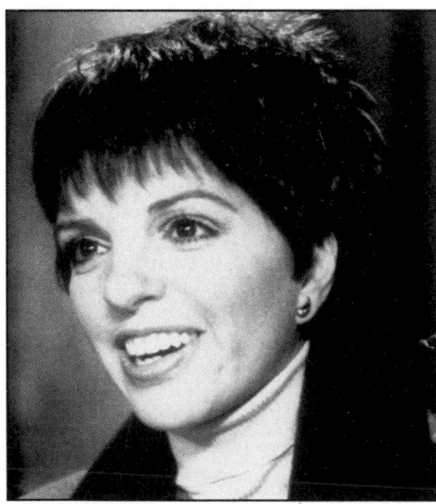

Liza Minnelli: No enemies!

The fourth is "punk" Pixie. This sounds like a contradiction in terms, and it is meant to be. This is the Pixie cut with a hard edge and threatening air about it. The best example of this look is worn by the fashion model Kristen McMenamy, who lends an air of menace to everything she does. This look has to be done perfectly to turn out right. If you end up mixing waif Pixie with punk Pixie the results are calamitous—it's a chance to end up looking like Dennis the Menace gone terribly, improbably

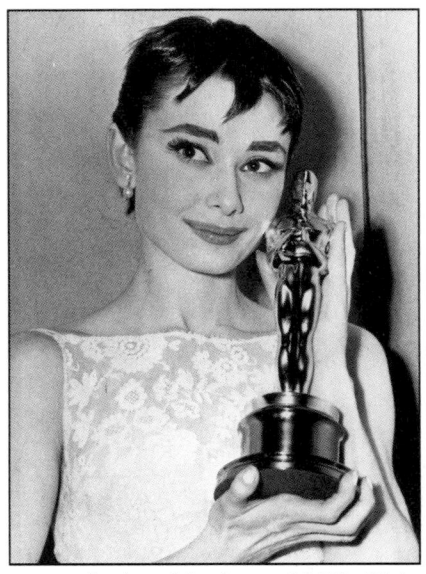

Audrey Hepburn: 1950s Pixie

wrong. Ironically, this version of the cut serves as a corrective for everything that is childlike, delicate and vulnerable about the rest of the Pixie's cuts. This Pixie comes right at you. As McMenamy wears it, this is one Pixie (and the only Pixie) people will cross the street to avoid.

There isn't much of a down-side to the Pixie, although people generally hate the name. "Pixie" strikes them as elfin and childish, as something out of the Brownies or a Disney film. It is likely that the name comes from Victorian children's books in which pixies wear a leaf bonnet on their heads. The points and shape of the leaf are roughly similar to the points and shape of the Pixie cut.[37] Both the name and the association are hopelessly old-fashioned. This look needs a new name.

The second problem is that the Pixie does not do "formal" very well. Unlike longer styles, which can be put up and adorned with combs and ribbons, the Pixie is pretty much a one-style cut. It looks acceptable on formal occasions, but it is hard to glamorize or formalize. You can "turn it up a little bit" by using styling products to give it a "super chic" edge. This is mostly a matter of making it look more sleek and more sharply defined. Or you can add hairpieces. But it is not easy to inflate and make grander and more mysterious.

The last problem is that the Pixie does not do "authority" very well. We would not, for instance, expect a woman running for office to wear one. Political office, some suppose, demands "helmet hair" of the kind worn by Margaret Thatcher. They insist that there is a good reason for the fact that we never saw a Pixie on Golda Meir, Kim Campbell, Benazir Bhuto or Elizabeth II. There may be something to this argument. Probably because of its youthful, waifish, ingenue quality, the Pixie may not always give a woman the *gravitas* she needs for public office.

On the other hand, Stella Rimington wears a Pixie, and this is a woman who knows a thing or two about power. Rimington is the head of MI-5, one of Britain's intelligence agencies. She has over two thousand employees and a budget of many millions of pounds. As Britain's spy master, Rimington is responsible for protecting Britain from international terrorism and the IRA. Perhaps Pixies are not so wrong for power positions after all.

The Historical Note

The Pixie has made several historical appearances. Something vaguely like it appeared after the French Revolution, when it was worn by aristocratic women either as an act of contrition or defiance, no one seems to know which. The look was called "*à la victime*," or "*à la sacrifice*." Hair was combed up from the neck, "leaving the neck bare," as historian Richard Corson ghoulishly puts it, "as if for the guillotine."[38]

Short hair was otherwise not welcome to the party. The eighteenth and nineteenth centuries generally seized upon women's hair as an opportunity for conspicuous consumption. Bigger was better. In this scheme, short hair was a confession of penury, an invitation for ridicule. It is not until the twentieth century that it established itself in North America.

The Pixie came to North America bearing chicness mostly because it was seen as European. It flourished particularly in the 1950s as a corrective, an antidote to the big hair enthusiasms of the moment. The Pixie emerged as an alternative, as a cut with its own very powerful meanings. Hollywood played a curious part in this. The dream machine has long

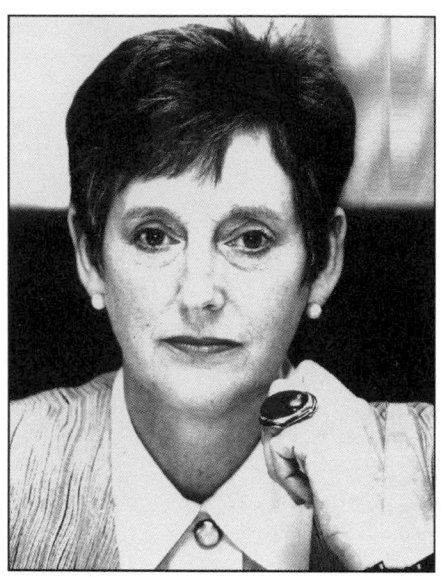

Stella Rimington: Spy-master Pixie

been a champion of big and blond hair, but it became a messenger of the Pixie look, perhaps in spite of itself, when it introduced Audrey Hepburn and Leslie Caron to American audiences.

Caron's introduction came in the 1951 film *An American In Paris*. She played the lover of an ex-GI who stayed on to pursue his art in a decayed Parisian garret. Caron and these romantic circumstances gave the look the *demi-monde* associations of the world of art. America was stunned. This was beauty on camera that had nothing to do with bigness or blondness. This was simply (and stunningly) chic.

Hepburn's introduction came a few years later in the 1954 film *Sabrina*. Playing a girl from the wrong side of the tracks, Hepburn's character returns from Paris with short hair and new confidence. Once again, the Pixie was presented as something coming from the Continent. And this time it was shown as something that could transform American women with devastating effect. Chalk up a second point for the Pixie.

But then the real fun began. Just one year after *Sabrina* there appeared a true '50s phenomenon. Her name was Françoise Sagan and she was the eighteen-year-old author of the novel *Bonjour Tristesse* (Good Morning, Sadness). The book was an unexpected hit, selling well in France and even better in America. *Life* interviewed Sagan and was wowed, reporting that "She likes to drive fast cars, use up the afternoons shooting dice for the drinks on cafe terraces, and spend whole evenings listening to jazz."[39] *Whole* evenings, mind you. To untutored American ears in the 1950s, listening to jazz, even a little jazz, was a statement of sophistication. Plainly, both the novelist (and her haircut) were the very picture of Parisian stylishness.

But the image of Sagan got even better. *Time* revealed that Sagan had written *Bonjour Tristesse* in a café in the shadow of the Sorbonne.[40] This settled it. In the 1950s, café life was *the* American idea of sophistication. It was worlds away from the suburban, car-centred, drive-in culture of the moment. And the idea of writing a novel in these circumstances completed the construction of Sagan (and her haircut) as perfectly, thrillingly exotic. It conjured the image of a young girl, fuelled by espresso and Gauloise, driven by creative demons, holding her head in her hands as she thought out the complexities of the novel inside her. Women raised in the Dick Van Dyke / Laura Petrie mode found this arresting and attractive. Here was a powerful alternative to the whole *Pillow Talk* / Doris Day scheme of things.

All this helped to confirm the image of the Pixie as something terribly, exquisitely, you know, kind of, *other*. The Pixie now stood for something outside the realm of the known and the usual. It was from another, wonderfully fashionable world. It helped to make up some of the aesthetic, emotional and stylistic deficits of 1950s American life.

The last Pixie proselytizer was Jean Seberg. Seberg starred in the 1959 film *Breathless*, directed by Jean-Luc

Godard, a man with impeccable avant-garde credentials. The intellectuals were satisfied that the film represented an important breakthrough. Not only was it experimental, it was hard to understand. Most important, it starred a beautiful young American who had forsworn Hollywood to make a career in the endlessly more creative and experimental circumstances of Europe.

Now we had a real-life heroine—not merely Hepburn playing at being an American in Paris, but a real American, really in Paris! Seberg was the completion of the fantasy. Here she was, an American who had claimed a place for herself in this exotic, avant-garde world with a haircut that captured all that was exotic and avant-garde about the place. The Pixie was now truly launched.

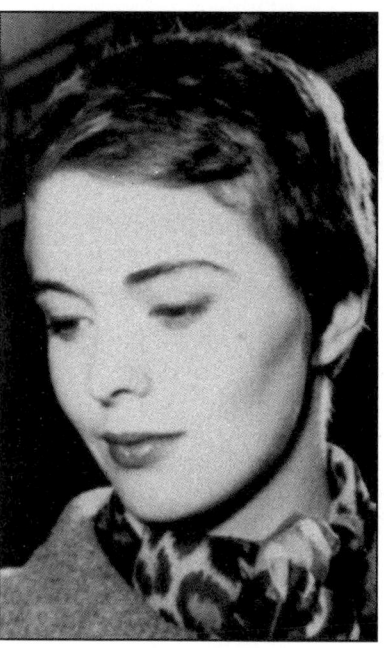

Seberg's Pixie

You couldn't have given America a more graceful learning curve. The Pixie was introduced to America in fully American films on the heads of relatively American stars. It then returned to America, this time in fully European films on the heads of relatively European stars. The Pixie, that strange and radical new look, came to America in gentle stages. Against all odds, in the face of big hair hegemony, America embraced it.

A decade later, another champion of the Pixie appeared in Europe. Twiggy came to stardom in the middle 1960s, her career carefully managed by a hairdresser named Justin de Villeneuve. Twiggy captured the gamine quality of the look almost perfectly. She appeared to the nation as a little girl who had lost her way and somehow

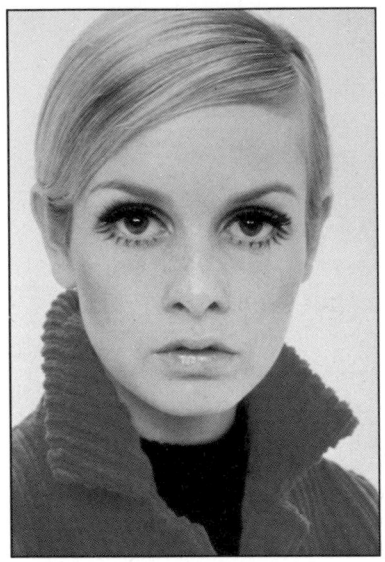

Twiggy's Pixie toppled Big Hair

ended up in a fashion photo shoot. Helene Gordon Lazareff, then editor of *Elle*, captured the universal reaction: "You say to yourself, 'Poor dear, I ought to take care of her.'"[41]

Twiggy's version of the Pixie is a difficult one because it was so utterly boyish. Twiggy seemed to paste her hair down so that it lost the charm of a traditional Pixie. But as the face (and hair) of the '60s, Twiggy did help to give new credibility to short hair at a time when many women continued to feel the siren call of long hair and big hair. Certainly, she helped to displace Jean Shrimpton, that massively famous and influential devotee of big hair.

Mia Farrow was also influential in the 1960s. The five-thousand-dollar haircut she got from Vidal Sassoon in preparation for *Rosemary's Baby* (1968) was an elegant Pixie (Sassoon tells us Farrow had been cutting it short well before[42]). The look actually figures in the movie. Farrow's character returns from the hairdresser and asks a horrified husband, "Do you like it? It's a Sassoon."

The Pixie appears to flourish at the beginning of every decade. It appeared early in the '50s, again early in the '60s and once more early in the '70s, '80s, and '90s.[43] Every decade is its own stylistic envelope—we expect it to transform us with new ideas and new images. But it often takes a decade three or four years to begin to define itself (it took the '60s almost five). So perhaps the Pixie appeals as a kind of "holding" look while we await our marching orders. The Pixie may flourish in this time of indeterminacy when Paris, Rome and Hollywood are still trying to make up their minds.

Linda Evangelista is famous for her short cut. She got it late in 1989, just as our "start of every decade" theory would have us expect. And she claims that she wanted it because she had "had enough of watching my haircut walk around everywhere." She wanted a "barbershop haircut ... like a little boy's," but she was horrified by the result. Had she risked too much? Would her career be damaged?

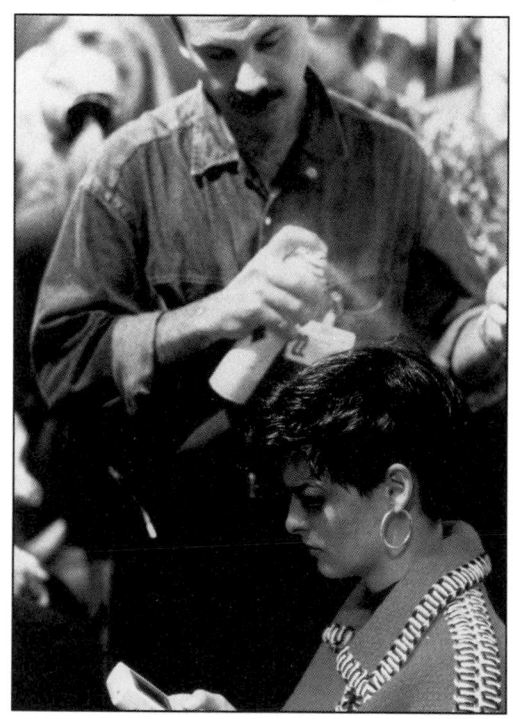

Within a couple of months, Evangelista appeared on all four *Vogue* covers: British, French, Italian and American. Short hair turned out to be a great career move. And much of the world followed suit. No doubt, Evangelista is once more seeing her haircut "walk around everywhere."

The Pixie cut is flourishing in the '90s. It conforms nicely to high fashion *and* to the sentiment against fashion. Designer Donna Karan sums up the

Linda Evangelista: Starting the new decade

virtues of the cut nicely: "Short hair is like a great dress. You just 'step into it' and go. Both simplify your life. And that is what the '90s are all about."[44]

In 1994, women started to move to short hair that is "hacked up, bleached blond or spiked with colour." Tina Gaudoin and Calvin Klein stylist Guido Palau believe this is part of the reaction against the 1980s: "Women are trying to look as fake as possible."[45] Whatever the 1990s and the next century hold for us, we will enter the future balanced precariously on the back of two very different circus ponies: anti-fashion naturalism and fashionable anti-naturalism.

The Pixie flourishes because it is fashionable and sophisticated on the one hand and hip and streetwise on the other. It is feminine and feminist. It is a fashion statement that has no exclusionary sting. It is elegant but agreeable. It is *à la mode* but it does not threaten or mock anyone. The Pixie holds the stage for many reasons, not the least of which is its ability to capture the contradictions of the moment and make them rather fetching.

The Minority Opinion

Men like the Pixie cut. It's companionable, attractive and unthreatening. Some of them, the knucklehead contingent, complain that there is nothing sexual about it. There is, as one of them put it, no "siren call." This is, of course, exactly what makes it so perfect for women who want to avoid "that certain kind of guy."

On the other hand, the Pixie does have a certain youthfulness, and this appeals to some men, again for the wrong reasons. The Pixie, in some male eyes, can be a sign of childlike dependency. But this is just the knucklehead brigade talking. Most men regard the look as professional, energetic, intelligent and forthright.

China Doll, Baby Doll or Cleopatra

- **What a stereotype—Asian women as delicate and passive!**
- **Cleopatra was a dominatrix!**

This look has several names: the "China Doll" the "Baby Doll" or sometimes the "Cleopatra" look. Each name has its own interpretation. When it's the "China Doll," it comes with stereotypic notions of the Asian female. It makes the wearer appear passive, delicate and dependent on men. Similar associations accompany the "Baby Doll": sweet, passive, needy. But when it's the Cleopatra look, it has another association altogether. Suddenly, it evokes a woman of power and of mystery. As the China or Baby Doll look, the cut is "cute." As the Cleopatra, it's "dramatic."

Respondents said this look has a seductive quality. There is, they said, something "beguiling" and "intriguing" about it, an air of mystery. These are the Asian and Egyptian associations speaking, probably. In spite of themselves, North Americans entertain romantic, nineteenth-century ideas about Asia and Egypt. In the stereotype, Asia is always "inscrutable" and Egypt "exotic." Both cultures become

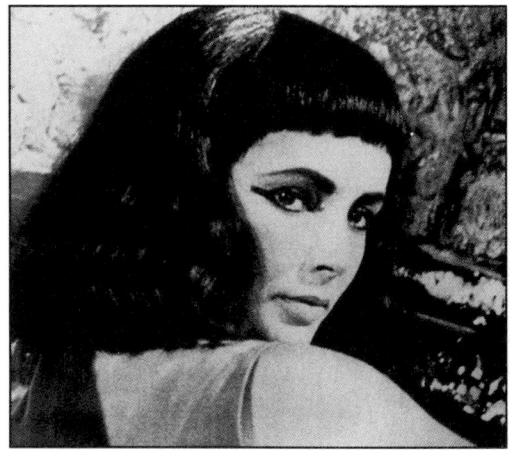

Liz Taylor's Cleopatra

staging grounds for fantasies of passive Asians and dominating Egyptians. Never mind that these ideas of Asia and Egypt are completely wrong, the look smoulders anyhow.

The Historical Note

This cut is a bob (one of several we review here), and it descends from the long and honourable bob tradition of the twentieth century. Louise Brooks, the 1920s film star, wore one. So did that other (and less well-known) star of the silent screen, Anna May Wong, and it may be from Ms. Wong that the "China Doll" association comes. On the strength of these associations, the look was immensely popular in the 1920s.

The sensational discovery in 1922-23 of King Tut's tomb delivered America into the hands of an Egyptian trend. Clothing, jewellery, footwear suddenly took on an Egyptian look. It is likely that hair was part of the trend.[46]

The 1920s were the time of the great bob rebellion. Women threw off the elaborate hairstyles of the last two centuries. The suffragette movement that swept North America, transforming voting privileges and clothing styles, also creat-ed pressure for a new look, for some-thing that cut away that great symbol of women's oppression, her "crowning glory." Women across the country went to men's barbershops and demanded to have their hair cut short.[47]

Ms. Chanel declared war on the ideas of Victorian finery

By the mid 1920s, the bob had taken on the impress of fashion. A music hall song from 1926 put the matter plainly:

> Sweet Susie Simpson had such lovely hair
> It reach'd down to her waist
> Till friends sweetly told her that around Mayfair
> Having hair was thought bad taste.
> "Bobb'd or shing-l'd it must be, dear,"
> said they,"if you wish to wed;"[48]

The China Doll was one of these new bobs. It was, to this extent, a refusal of women's subordinate status and her role as ornament. But it was also freighted with sexist notions of who a woman was. The China Doll was simulta-neously a blow for freedom and a declaration of depen-dence. Perhaps it takes some of its mystery (and ambiva-lence) from this founding contradiction.

Coco Chanel's haircut was a kind of bob. And what else would we expect? Coco Chanel harboured a great hostility for the traditional roles of femaleness. She aston-ished polite society by striding around in the riding pants of her lover, Boy Capell. (No, he was not still wearing them.) Through her fashion design, Ms. Chanel declared war on the ideas of Victorian finery, on women as delicate pieces of porcelain, on style as the woman's golden cage. It was inevitable that a woman of her standing would adopt the rebellious bob. But she is not, in fact, the inventor of the bob. She came to it relatively late and only because of a household accident that required her to cut her hair short. (The fashion designer Poiret is credited with having invented the bob in 1917.)[49]

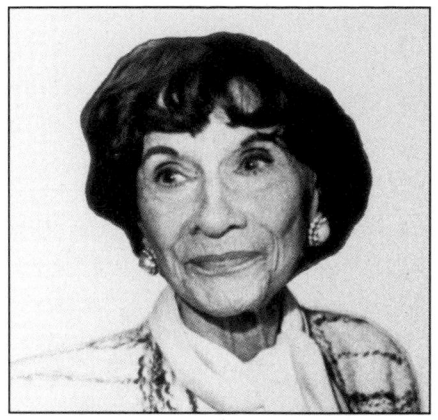

Coco Chanel: Rebellious Bob

Since the 1920s, the haircut has enjoyed two moments in the sun. It was worn by Elizabeth Taylor in the 1963 movie phenomenon *Cleopatra* and, as a result of this blockbuster, it rose to fashion and widespread adoption in the 1960s.[50] And it is enjoying a certain vogue in the 1990s: it made a recent and memorable performance in the recent Michael Jackson video "Remember the Time."

The Minority Opinion

Men report finding this cut attractive and sometimes a little intimidating. They are responding, no doubt, to the passive and dominating aspects of the look's symbolism. Men also noted seeing a kind of mystery in the cut. Who is this woman? What is she thinking? Can she by relied upon to do the predictable thing? Is she inhabited by instincts and inclinations that are strange and foreign? This haircut, associated as it is with exotic, faraway places, made some men wonder whether the wearer might not be motivated by the exotic and the far away. This cut gave them pause. It caught their attention.

The Mature Bob

- This is really the beginning of the end, isn't it.
- I think this looks great on her!

It's almost a law in our culture: as a woman ages, she shall cut her hair. Long hair until college; short hair afterwards. I noticed this years ago when I sat listening to a museum lecture so dull as to pass all comprehension. To amuse myself I began looking at the haircuts of the women in the audience. Every woman under twenty-five had long hair, and every woman over forty had short hair. The women in between appeared to be in transition.

Research for this book confirmed the pattern. While there are lots of exceptions (not the least of which is a current fashion for short hair for woman in their twenties and thirties), women (and hairdressers) told me over and over again that as they grew older they cut their hair shorter. This rule has several implications, none of them particularly fair or just. Traditionally, women who are in their sixties and seventies are ridiculed if they have long hair (unless they wear it up). They are called hags and crones. Women in their fifties who have long hair are seen to be fighting age. Women in their forties are seen to be holding out.

It's almost a law in our culture: as a woman ages, she shall cut her hair

Thus speaks the stereotype. Gloria Steinem wears longish hair with impunity, but then she is working to reinvent everything we think about women.

There is a tyranny at work here. No woman told me that she liked saying goodbye to her hair—she was cutting it because she didn't want to appear to be "frivolous," or "vain," or, gulp, "ageing badly." She was not cutting her hair because she wanted to. She was cutting it because she had to.

There is no good explanation for this pattern. It does, however make for a striking rite of passage. Several hairdressers told me that they prepare their clients for the "big haircut" with care and caution. Often they see the occasion coming well before the client, and they make it their job to ease the transition, to get the client ready for this shift into maturity. Some hairdressers even have a kind of wake for long hair before it's cut. It is, say the hairdressers and the clients, a sad farewell to youth.

Some people are persuaded that the move to shorter hair is driven by changes that take place as a woman ages. They insist that the face changes shape and is sometimes less well suited to longer hair. And that the quality of the hair also changes, becoming more brittle and less vital. All of this demands, they claim, shorter hair.

This argument has some substance. Important changes do take place. Grey hair does have a different, coarser texture. Older hair does have less body and shine. But it is also true that we are now very sophisticated in our abilities to keep hair healthy and to repair it when damaged. Sometimes, however, the deterioration in the quality of hair is not the work of nature but nurture. It is a lifetime of bad treatment that damages hair until there is no recourse but to cut it short. And the cycle continues. Bad treatment demands progressively shorter cuts until women are left with a "Brillo pad" effect.

The move to short hair is not a necessity, demanded of us by advancing years and ageing hair. For the real explanation for this pattern we need to look a little deeper.

Shorter hair has become a way of signalling that a woman has put the vanities and preoccupations of youth behind her

One respondent had an interesting explanation. "Men like long hair [on a woman]. And as a woman gets older and gets married and has kids, she comes out of circulation. That's why she cuts her hair. These women aren't out to make any big impressions." By this thoroughly male-centred account, women cut their hair short because they are no longer "in the market."

In many western cultures, it was customary in past generations for women to signify their virginity with long, flowing tresses and to wear this hair up after marriage. In contemporary culture, women of a certain age cut it, whether or not they are married. They move to short hair as a marker of their own maturity and not because they are someone's wife. All of this may be an indicator of sexual access, but more probably, shorter hair has become a way of signalling that a woman has put the vanities and preoccupations of youth behind her. In our culture, shorter hair is a way of saying "I am getting on with life."

It is also possible that sometimes these cuts are a retreat from fashion. As some women begin to cut their hair shorter, they care less about the kinds of cuts they get. These shorter cuts get mixed reviews. While some see them as perfectly suitable for the world of work, others see them as insufficiently fashionable and equivalent to sequined T-shirts, tight, acid-washed jeans and ankle bracelets.

Still others called this a classic look for middle age. They said it was attractive but not especially fashionable. "Presentable but not very presentable," was the way one person put it. People talked about this style as being "handsome." And this is a way of saying the cut transcends "girlish" flips and elaborations. It is a serious cut for a serious person—good-looking and, more particularly, dignified. It was seen to be a good cut for ageing gracefully. "This is the haircut grandmothers are supposed to have: nice, short and manageable." In general, the mature bob is not considered to be especially upscale. It is seen to be out of the buzz of fashion. One women called it "predictable." Another called it "boring." This is the right cut for the age, my respondents seemed to be telling me, but it is probably the only cut for the age. It was to this extent not so much a choice as an obligation.

The Historical Note

These are all bobs of a kind. They are heirs to that great twentieth century tradition of the bob in which women threw off the extravagances of Victorian hair. Short hair was suddenly the sign of women who wished to control their own lives. It was a sign of women who wished to get out from under the role of ornament. The tradition continues.

But women are also variously mirroring, quoting and borrowing short haircuts worn by men. Take, for instance, our first cut. This has both a duck's tail in the back and a falling curl in the front. Both of these were favoured by men in the 1950s. The ducktail, or DA (for "Duck's Ass"), was invented by Mexican teenagers who wore zoot suits. Why the young men of Mexico were suddenly overwhelmed by the need to look like mallards now escapes us, but we do know that teenage males everywhere were immediately impressed. Once the look had been popularized by Tony Curtis, Elvis and James Dean, it spread quickly. It even found its way to England where it was adopted by the Teddy Boys, the first official "teenagers" in Britain.

Several of these aficionados of the DA also wore the falling curl or "quiff" in front. Elvis was the one who made it popular. The audience would wait with sexual anticipation for the moment when his quiff would break loose from its moorings and begin to swing wildly from side to side. This look is still popular among men and was worn by rockabilly bands like the Stray Cats and by Japanese Teddy Boys.[51]

Plainly, the male version of this look is devoted to the advertisement of male sexuality. Women who wear it play out messages of their own. There is a message of open sexuality about this cut, and this is probably what gives the look its "low-class" character in certain eyes.

The Minority Opinion

Men are not especially generous with this hair. But what they do get from it is an "I'm married" message: "This one went shorter because she's got a mate but she still wants to stay a little wild." One man went so far as to say that you wanted your wife to have a cut like this: "Otherwise, other men are going to be hitting on her all the time." For these men, short hair is a marker of marital status. Isn't it a little strange that men do not change *their* hair after marriage?

This cut was also seen to be a strategic move: "She doesn't want to be judged by her hair. She wants everything else to do the talking." There is a rough-and-ready kind of feminism about this comment. This man is saying he is no longer supposed to respond only sexually, he is prepared to attend to other aspects of a woman's character. Finally!

This testimony suggests that short haircuts are wise choices for women who find our present gender stereotypes oppressive. They send a very clear message and tell men that sexist sexual overtures are not welcome.

The Blunt Cut

- This is the perfect cut for the 1980s, the *only* cut for the 1980s
- This goes with those broad-shouldered suits
- It looks so smart

This look is highly attractive and entirely current, but its heyday was the 1980s. It emerged as the single best cut for women to wear as they sought a place in the corporate world. The look became (and remains) a signature look of the professional woman, the very picture of competence and seriousness. And it worked! Women carried it into the corporate world, into the boardroom, the law courts, the operating theatre. The blunt cut did (and does) its work with all the professionalism and competence of the women who wore it. What this look was designed to do was to send men a clear message: "I am here as your colleague, I am here as your equal, I can do what you can do (and I can probably do it better)."

The great fear of the '80s was that men would react to the presence of women in the workplace by asking them to go for coffee, that they would be so aroused or threatened by "skirts" in the workplace that they would be incapable of giving women their due. Women needed a way of declaring their intentions and the "dress for success" look fit the bill perfectly. It was standardized, high contrast, broad-shouldered, a little severe and perfectly disciplined. It said, "Put aside your stereotypes about women being flighty, emotional and undependable; women are ready for the demands of the corporate world."

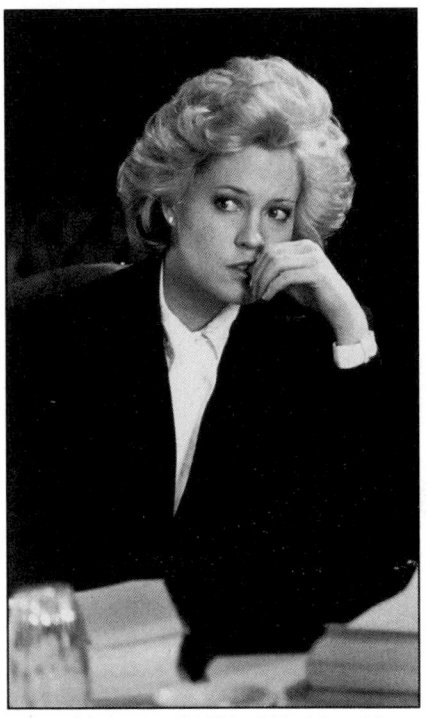

Melanie Griffith: Working blunt

Enter the blunt cut. It was symbolically everything the "dress for success" look was. It had the same standardized, severe, disciplined character to it. Plus it looked stunning with the broad-shouldered suits of the moment. The clear, broad line of the shoulders was repeated in the clear, broad line of the cut. Here was a haircut that could, and would, get the job done.

Traditionally, women's hair has been long and flowing. Visually, it makes a symbolic connection between her head and her body. The sensuality of the body reaches up into the head; the passions of the mind reach down into the body. The blunt cut stopped all this. Just at a time when women needed to say, "Observe, I am a creature of reason and objectivity" to their sexist colleagues, the blunt cut emerged to show a stark contrast between the head and the body. The blunt cut declared them separate. The blunt cut *made* them separate.

This look was perfect for Brenda, that legal paragon of efficiency we met in Chapter Two. Everything about

Brenda spoke of her abilities. The blunt cut and the Chanel suit spoke as one.

So completely did the blunt cut capture female executives that the corporate world suddenly had a new class distinction: executive women wore the blunt cut while secretaries continued to wear sexual clothing and high hair. This was the great visual theme of the film *Working Girl*, the story of one woman's move up the corporate ladder. Melanie Griffith has a smart new haircut—not quite a blunt cut, but close. Her secretary friends have unbelievably high hair.

This is not to say that the corporate woman of the 1980s was not sexual. She was frequently utterly sexual. But there was a clear message in place: "Let us attend to the affairs of the world, before we consider those of the heart."

Some women complain that the blunt cut that works so well at work does not work especially well at home. Children, one mother told me, react to its severity. It does not have the softness "Mommy" is supposed to have.

The blunt cut has several variations. Some women add volume by using perms, rollers or blow-dryers, and this gives the blunt a certain bigness. Fat blunts can be very effective. They demand attention without appearing to request it. They can manage to be both severe and voluptuous all at once. Blunts can also be bevelled so that the hair on the outside of the cut is longer. This lets the blunt mix severity with grace. In both cases, blunt variations capture a perfectly professional look and smuggle in a certain sensuality or softness in the process. Fat and feathered blunts let the wearer have her cake and eat it too.

The Historical Note

The blunt cut is a classic bob. It is part of that great tradition that begins in the 1920s. And it is driven by the same spirit of feminist revolution: "Do not ask us to wear hair that declares our gender and compromises our place in the world."

A later influence was perhaps the "pageboy." This look was worn by Ginger Rogers, Greta Garbo, June Allyson and Grace Kelly. It had roughly the same silhouette as the blunt and some of its simplicity of line. The characteristic "turn under" of the pageboy was antithetical to the blunt, but otherwise the pageboy may be the blunt's ancestor.[52]

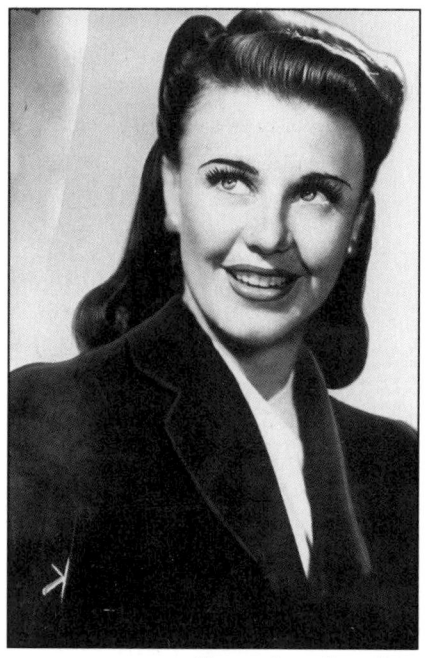

Ginger in a Pageboy

The blunt cut owes most to the revolution accomplished by Vidal Sassoon in the 1960s. It follows Sassoon's first principle: the shape of the hair must come from the shape of the cut. And it is a thoroughly Sassoon cut to the extent that it refuses the teasing, fussing and the ornamental labour that decorative cuts demand.

The Minority Opinion

Most men say they get the intended message of this cut loud and clear. The hair tells them that the wearer wants men to honour her as a colleague before they respond to her sexuality. But it is a difficult cut for sexist men. It is severe and precise just where and when they want women to be soft and yielding. Their reaction is one of confusion and even hostility.

Other men merely find this a "practical" cut. It is the kind of cut worn by women who have "married and settled down." It says they are no longer creatures of vanity and sensuality. They have embraced the imperatives of middle age. They are getting on with their lives. So say my respondents.

The 1990s Career Coif

- **This looks really polished, really professional**
- **This is the look of the 1990s**

The "career coif" is to the '90s what the blunt cut was to the '80s. It is the cut that for many women best defines who they are and where they stand. (It says something about the difference between the two decades that the blunt cut should have been so, well, blunt, while the career coif is so much higher, softer and fuller.) The career coif is now at the height of its popularity.

This cut has come to prominence for a couple of reasons. First, by the end of the '80s, it was generally decided

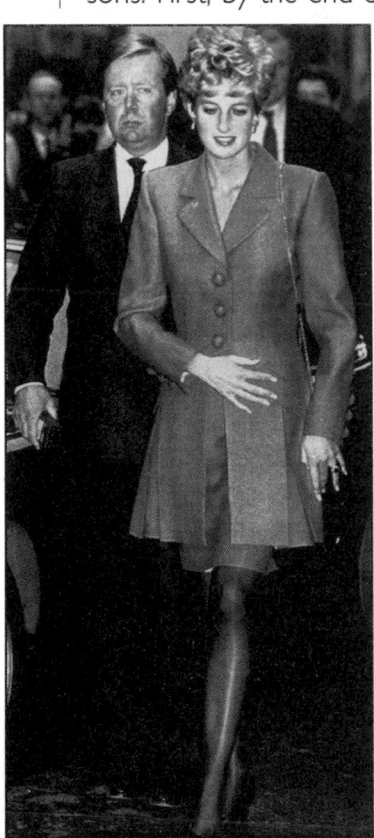

that women had established a place for themselves in the corporate world. The war was won. Padded shoulders, monochromatic suits and the blunt cut were no longer necessary. It was time to move on.

Women wanted a look that retained an '80s discipline but that now also had a '90s imagination and freedom. They were *not* quite ready for wild and wonderful hair. Except in the most creative workplaces this was still unacceptable. But they did want something that breathed, something with scale and motion. They wanted something that loosened up without coming undone. And so this cut was born.

But there was a second strategy at work. Women also wanted hair that spoke about

Princess Diana: In a Career Coif   their special powers in the world of work. As one career woman told me, "People are looking to women for vision and imagination. So it's okay to have hair that's a little bit sexy and powerful. A bit of flamboyance is okay." We've come a long way since the '80s or, as another respondent put it, "Around here, women with severe haircuts are being classified as order-takers, as analysts; not the leaders." The career coif became the new mark of leadership.

It takes some conjuring to figure out why this cut should be so perfect for women of the world of work. One woman told me that, in order to qualify, the new cut had to steer a careful course through all the aesthetic and cultural possibilities out there. To succeed as the new look it could not be too ornate, artsy, flip, funky or old-fashioned.

"Ornate" is a problem because you can't overdress for work without looking like a "fuss pot" or something "too decorative to get any work done." "Artsy" is a problem because you want people to be creative but not too creative. "Flip" and "funky" are problems because the corporate world will tolerate only so much irreverence. "Old-fashioned" is a problem because it says you are not in touch with the dynamism of a quickly changing corporate world. The career coif is well designed for the world of work.

This look is also seen to have a certain "polish," one of the crucial ingredients of success in the fast lane. Polish is a statement of self-confidence, of class and finally of style. It says that a woman is a striding, powerful, graceful presence in the world of work. Polish is a kind of quiet charisma, a quality that works well in the world of work.

The '90s has been declared a decade that cares about simplicity, that refuses elaborateness, that turns it's back on '80s sumptuousness. Katie Couric, co-host of the "Today" show, has even called it the decade of the "plain chick." But the career coif is not a "plain chick" cut.[53] It is elaborate, labour intensive and a little bit grand. The rest of the '90s may be marching to a simpler tune, but the fashion in corporate hair is listening to a drummer of its own. It is leaving the nervous, narrow parameters of the 1980s and expanding with new expressiveness, authority, grace and style.

The Historical Note

This cut has a long and distinguished history, and it has made several appearances in the history of hair. Ava Gardner wore it in 1950. In 1954, it made the cover of *Life* magazine as "the Italian cut."[54] In 1958, *Vogue* praised a variation called the "firecracker pouf" for its "careless charm."[55] Marilyn Monroe wore a variation of this cut in the 1950s. Her adoption made it mainstream and gave it charisma.

The look reappeared in 1964 as the new haircut of one of the great models of the period, Suzy Parker. Until this cut, Parker had always worn her hair long and full. The world of fashion was taken aback at the change. *Vogue* said she looked like "a curl-wreathed head of the Mercury that was found in the ruins of a Hadrian edifice."[56]

This cut is also being worn by the former Guess Jeans model Anna Nicole Smith, who deliberately styled herself after Marilyn Monroe. Whitney Houston adopted it fairly early. And the most famous recruit is Princess Di. (Aristocrats may no longer set the fashion, but when they follow it, so do many others.)

The look established itself with a vengeance in 1990 when it was adopted by what seemed like all of Hollywood, including Madonna, Geena Davis, Daryl Hannah and Linda Evangelista.[57] By September 1991, it was being declared the look of choice for professional working women. Image consultants in New York City were recommending shorter, fuller hair: "Your hair reflects your managerial power. I believe that longer hair equals less power because the emphasis is on your hair, not your abilities or intelligence."[58]

From the heads of 1950s movie stars to the heads of women in the '90s career world: the corporate coif has come a long way.

The Minority Opinion

Men are generally impressed with this look. They find it attractive and appealing. This look exudes a certain sexuality.

But men also find it a little intimidating. They can see the self-possession. They know this is a cut with power. Partly, this has to do with the way women are *wearing* this cut. Their manner is forthright and self-confident, and the cut comes to carry the same message. For some men, it's all a bit puzzling. The cut is sexual—it has a Marilyn Monroe echo—but the demurring, subordinate behaviour is missing. They are not quite sure what to make of it.

Men see this as a fashionable cut, and that makes it puzzling, too. Fashion is, generally, a source of mystery for males. It is, after all, only *style*, and therefore always a substitute for substance. But they *do* know that style can make them ridiculous. They know that if they stray too far from fashion, no one (not even other men) will take them seriously. Generally, men treat fashion the way bears treat electricity: it is not something they understand completely but it is something they've come to respect.

Shaved and Shorn

- It's ugly, it's masculine, she wants to be spotted
- You need real beauty and confidence to pull this off
- She's wearing her inner suffering on her head
- Sometimes a girl's got to do what a girl's got to do
- It makes me feel so free!

"Shaved and Shorn" is a look to love or hate. It is, after all, a political statement, one that says, "I dislike your world. I refuse it." Those who love it say the look is a tough, honourable way of taking a stand. Those who hate it say the look is self-dramatizing, self-righteous

Would O'Connor wear this cut if she didn't happen to look like Audrey Hepburn?

and really irritating. One of them told me, "I think it's just another way of saying 'F**k you.'" The wearer is content whatever the reaction. She welcomes friends and expects enemies.

Politics aside, the look takes confidence. Not everyone can wear it well. Sigourney Weaver managed it in *Alien 3*. Kirstie Alley wore it in *Star Trek II: The Wrath of Khan*. (What is it about outer space that makes us believe women will suddenly go hairless?) And Sinead O'Connor has worn it most of her career. But all three begin with large eyes and fine features.

Sinead O'Connor may wear it to *emphasize* her beauty. "Look," she says in effect, "other women need their hair to make them beautiful. Not me." The radical gesture is, perhaps, an act of vanity. It comes down to this: would O'Connor wear this cut if she didn't happen to look like Audrey Hepburn?

There is a kinder interpretation, of course. O'Connor and other wearers want us to know they are refusing conventional ways of thinking about women. They believe conventional haircuts are so deeply embedded in a sexist culture that they cannot be worn without compromising the wearer's identity. Siouxsie Sioux ("Susie Sue"), the English rock star, took this position early in her career. Before she became the goddess of Goth, she cut her hair very short. "I've always tried to be the antithesis of the curvy, tanned, blond bombshell."[59] For her, the shorn look has been a useful ideological tool.

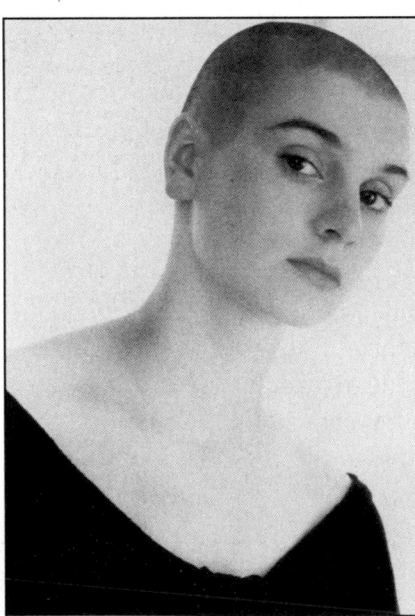

Sinead O'Connor: Shaved and Shorn

This position is hard to take issue with. Every look in this chapter is charged with a certain conventional idea of femaleness. If you don't happen to subscribe to these ideas, you're in an awkward spot. Your hair betrays you. Any haircut says you accept the status quo. For some people, there is only one solution: you must get rid of your hair. Some women wear the shaved and shorn look not because of what it is. They wear it because of what it isn't.

But some women react *against* the protest message. "Listen," they told me with feeling, "I can be feminine and feminist." For them, the shorn look is hostile and provocative. It forces a suspicion. If this is the way you feel about *your* femaleness, what are you saying about *my* femaleness? And who are you to comment on how I see myself as a woman?

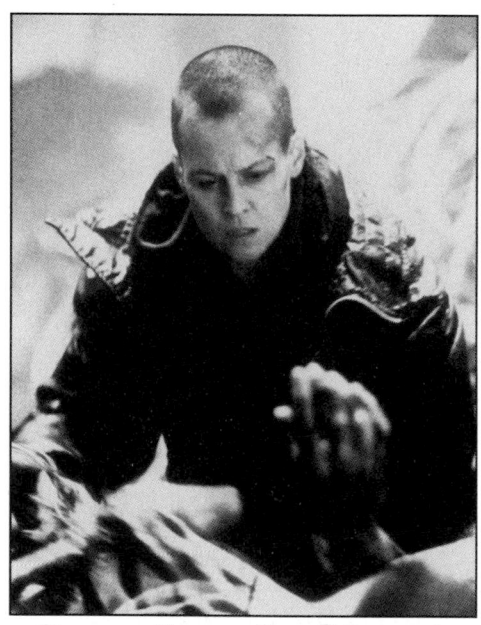

Sigourney Weaver: Shaved for stardom

The Historical Note

Very short hair has put in relatively few appearances in the history of hair. Joan of Arc is supposed to have used it to declare her uncompromising spirit. It appears again on the head of one of the mistresses of Charles VII of fourteenth-century France. In the 1920s, the Russian poet Vladimir Mayakovsky used the cut to promote his work.[60] And it was used in the 1940s by the Resistance to punish French women who collaborated with the Nazis. In the 1950s, women wore a "feminine butch" in imitation of the male brush cut.[61] In the 1960s, the Parisian designer Jacques

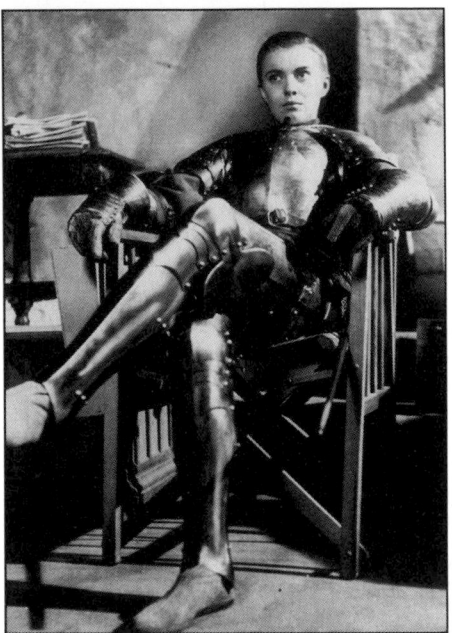

Hollywood's Joan of Arc in a Shaved and Shorn

Esterel had his models shaved, declaring, "Women are imprisoned by their own hair."[62]

Punks have worn the look with enthusiasm. (Sinead O'Connor still gets notes from punks who believe she must be one of them. "I tell them to sod off."[63]) Skinheads use the look to declare their hostility for hippie self-indulgence. In the process, they have managed to give it a certain jack-booted infamy.[64] The look is enjoying growing popularity among men, especially as a result of the influence of the lords of the basketball court, Charles Barkley and Michael Jordan.[65] It's too early to tell whether this version of the look will cross gender boundaries. Several models now wear the look for their own reasons, and this bodes well. (Sometimes Paris can do what Hollywood can't.)

The Minority Opinion

Predictably, many men are threatened by this look. They are so accustomed to seeing women in terms of their hair, they are a little confused when they're given nothing to go on. Some of them are quick to suppose the wearer must be a lesbian. The logic is: "Women wear hair to please us. If they cut off their hair, it must be because they don't want to please us, and this can only mean that they are gay." This is the usual sexist nonsense.

Perfect Strangers, Perfect Friends:
Myths and Realities in the
Hairdresser-Client Relationship

*I*nventing the world of hair is almost impossible to do alone. Generally, it takes two: a woman and her hairdresser. There are, after all, literally hundreds of cut and colour combinations, and thousands of executable selves. Finding the one that will have real transformational effect demands a long and substantial partnership.

The hairdresser-client relationship is never easy. When it works, it's extraordinary: hairdresser and client care the world for one another; they work in perfect tandem; they become, of necessity, deeply embedded in one another's emotional lives. But more typically the relationship is difficult, delicate and changeable. Communication breaks down

> *Hairdressers: vain, superficial, temperamental and wilful*

frequently. Trust and intimacy never materialize. The relationship glints with constant promise but never really seems to get anywhere. Perfect friends remain, mostly, perfect strangers.

For some poor souls the relationship between hairdresser and client is an exercise in misery. Try as they may, they succeed only in inventing new ways of frustrating one another. The salon becomes a battlefield, the encounter between hairdresser and client a constant clash of wills.

The problem is that the relationship is riddled with myths and misconceptions. Hairdressers and their clients struggle to make contact across a barrier of ignorance and misunderstanding. We have, it turns out, an amazing number of suspicions about hairdressers. They are supposed to be vain, superficial, temperamental and wilful. Most are modern-day myths, falsehoods raised to the status of a commonplace. And what dangerous myths they are! It is hard to imagine a more toxic or more slanderous brew.

Clients: arbitrary, wilful, peculiar and rude

Hairdressers have reciprocal doubts and misconceptions. From their side of the chair, clients can appear arbitrary, wilful, peculiar and rude. As I began to document these hostilities, I began to feel I was talking to the former citizens of East and West Berlin. There is an astonishing legacy of suspicion, rumour, backbiting and hard-line animosity here. Hairdressers don't understand clients any better than clients understand them.

My objective in this chapter is to cast myself as a kind of Henry Kissinger, to bring both parties to the bargaining table that they might work out some more stable, more comprehending and more successful relationship. And the first step in a workable peace is to sort through the myths and realities of the hairdresser-client relationship. It's time to clear the air and start anew.

Myths of Hairdressing

Stereotypes are like old slippers—they may look like hell, but they feel so wonderful we are loath to part with them. The fact that they are utterly wrong does not discourage us. After all, they confirm our favourite and most deep-seated prejudices. They reassure us that the world is just as it should be. We *like* thinking them. We like thinking them so much, nothing I say will likely make us stop. But I'm going to try.

- Myth number one: Hairdressers are not very bright. Who would do something as "unimportant" as cutting hair when you could be designing buildings, addressing the Supreme Court or performing brain surgery? No one does hair by choice. They do it, the myth says, because they can't do anything else. The attitude is summed up in the words of a twenty-five-year-old hair-dresser from Toronto: "'Oh look, there's another thing she can't do. It's off to hair school with her.' It was hair-dressing for girls and mechanics for boys."

    Hidden in this is the further myth that hairdressing is the work of a simpleton. Anybody can do it; just about anybody does. This is not rocket science, high finance or air-traffic control. The term "profession" is, of course, right out of the question, and even the term "craft"

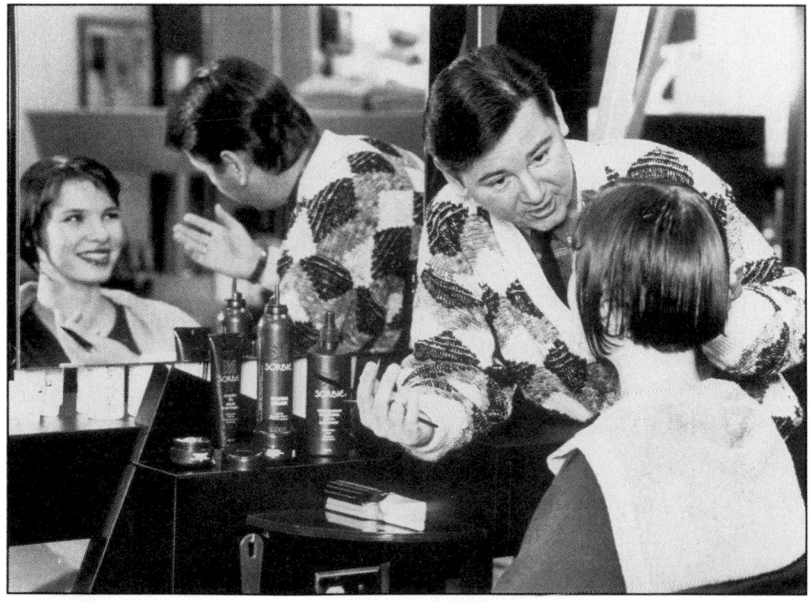

Mental health agents with cuts and curls

implies more difficulty and discipline than properly applies. Hairdressing is a "trade," and even this term threatens to dignify the enterprise. Hairdressing is *easy*.

- Myth number two: Hairdressers are superficial. There is a logical argument for this one. Hair doesn't count for anything. Serious people do not care about it. Therefore anyone who is drawn to the superficial must be superficial (according to the principle that like attracts like).

But it's not just hair that's unimportant. The larger world of fashion is unimportant, too. Clothing, interior design, hair, make-up—these things comprise the realm of the ridiculous, a woman's world in which one senseless fad is continually replaced by another. Fashion has no rhyme or reason. It is a giddy, shapeless, senseless swirl. In our culture, fashion concerns itself with the superficial. It *is* the superficial.

Literally, this is true. The term "superficial" comes from the latin word for "surfaces," and hair, make-up, clothing and the world of fashion are all, to be sure, surfaces of contemporary life. But western (and especially northern European and New World) cultures harbour a hostility for these surfaces. Westerners are most inclined to believe

Myth number five: Hairdressers have personalities deformed by vanity

that surfaces are a playground for dishonesty, deception and glibness. It is westerners especially who fear, mock and devalue them. Not all cultures see superficial things with quite the same distrust and loathing as our own. Indeed, this is one of our civilization's defining characteristics.

This western hostility for fashion is evident everywhere in the world of hair. The late film critic and writer Jay Scott captured it in a short story. Here a hairdresser describes his colleagues:

Sean's got great teeth and a great earring and a great LOOK that just looks different every week, Sean's LOOK is Giorgio Armani Uomo Vogue today and Ralph Lauren Coors Beer tomorrow, but tasteful, toujours tasteful, and Liz ... has got a great LOOK, too, I mean of course she does, she has a nose jewel.[1]

   Slaves of fashion, heads filled with passing fancies: hairdressers are, according to this myth, silly creatures drifting in a world utterly bereft of substance or, those crucial Protestant properties, gravity and ballast.

• Myth number three: Hairdressers are from lower-class families. "Good" families send their children into law, medicine and dentistry, not into hairdressing. You only go into hairdressing when your alternative is blue-collar labour. One hairdresser told me it took him ten years to tell new acquaintances what he did. This is customary. Hairdressing is seen to be the refuge for people from the "wrong" side of town.

• Myth number four: Hairdressers exhibit an exaggerated sexuality. The myth says that hairdressers are either foppishly gay or promiscuously heterosexual. In one case, the male hairdresser is a "flaming queer." In the other, he is a sexual philanderer, sleeping with as many clients as he can (like the Warren Beatty character in the film *Shampoo*). In either case, hairdressers are beyond the pale of "conventional" (i.e., monogamous heterosexual) sexuality. (Remember the knowing conspiratorial smirk that Cynthia and Bernard share when they see Lawrence's black eye: "Too much fun last night, Lawrence?")

• Myth number five: Hairdressers have personalities deformed by vanity. *Time* magazine captured (and helped to perpetuate) the myth in 1965 when it described the typical hairdresser as someone who is "vain, fickle, unreliably charming and dependably indiscreet [as well as] never too far from a mirror to lose sight of himself."[2]

- Myth number six: Hairdressers are unstable. The hairdresser can do brilliant work but he is, finally, at the mercy of his emotions. According to this stereotype, hairdressers have that "high strung" temperament of the creative individual. They are, like wilful children or manic depressives, "explosive."

- Myth number seven: Hairdressers are the captives of a cruel and relentless game of status competition. They delight in wounding clients, staff and one another. They trade endlessly in vicious gossip. They delight in "bitchy" remarks. And nothing hurts them more, or destabilizes them faster, than being the object of someone else's gossip. The stereotype says hairdressers live and die by small, keenly fought skirmishes in a relentless status game.

- Myth number eight: Hairdressers are inclined to be self-dramatizing. They are little Oscar Wildes. They do not speak, they declaim. They do not stand, they posture. They do everything with a flourish, the better to draw attention to themselves. Alternatively, they bully in the manner of a latter day Napoleon. They are insufferably conceited and expect the world to bend itself to their will. They are happiest when barking bad-tempered orders at clients and staff. These hairdressers, says the myth, are constantly "acting out."

Whew! Our stereotypes insist that the hairdresser has no class credentials, limited intelligence, performs a virtually worthless task, labours as the prisoner of fashion, and is subject to defects of every kind, including sexual excess, personality deformations, arrogance and status anxiety. My, my, my. We have not been kind.

Plainly, any one of these myths is enough to blunt a client's confidence in the transformational abilities of her hairdresser — not to mention, a hairdresser's confidence in him (or her) self. Together, they disqualify the hairdresser from serious consideration. They so diminish the hairdresser that we are unprepared to trust them with the selves they might otherwise transform.

Myths of Hairdressing from the Inside

Needless to say, hairdressers, generally, do not believe our myths about them. But they have not, on the whole, made things better. They have not given us a more accurate or honest account of who they are and what they do. Instead, they have muddied the waters by creating several stereotypes of their own and, sometimes, by confirming our preconceptions by acting them out.

Hairdressers like to compare themselves to a variety of other groups: doctors, priests, artists, rock stars. Ernest Adler, the great American hairdresser, liked to argue that a visit to the hairdresser was worth six trips to the psychiatrist. And there is some justice to this comparison. In fact, as we shall see, clients do look to their hairdressers for psychological counsel. A good hairdresser is skilled at reading his or her client, good at probing for the root of an unhappiness. The really good ones give wonderfully deft, subtle and effective advice.

> *We were, as a group, walking towards the swirling fury of sound and light as if programmed from birth to do so*

Several hairdressers I interviewed compared themselves to medical doctors, saying, "We're the only other profession that's allowed to touch people." These hairdressers believe their touch has a healing quality, and they have plenty of proof that this is so. Over and over, they have seen the transformation that an hour at the salon can work upon a client.

Hairdressers also compare themselves to rabbis and priests. They have told me over and over again that the chair is a kind of confessional and that the client uses his or her time with the hairdresser to unburden the soul: "My clients can't talk to anyone the way they talk to me." And so it is. Hairdressers acknowledge and absolve. They listen and forgive. They cut away hair. They cut away guilt.

Hairdressers also compare themselves to artists. The great Antoine believed that there was no difference between his work in plaster and his work in hair. In both cases, he was sculpting heads. Next to the medical comparison, this is perhaps the favourite myth hairdressers like to tell one another about themselves.

And finally, some hairdressers style themselves as rock-and-roll stars. I saw this at a recent hair show. We were all crowded around the stage watching master stylists work. The woman at the podium was saying: "… and I think you notice that we have a very different look this year. We decided that the '90s are a time for going back to basics. This year we are emphasizing training and quality. No smoke and mirrors this year." Everyone nodded piously. For this was the new decade, and, yes, we had put smoke and mirrors behind us. One of the stylists stepped forward and told us he now buys clothes to last several years instead of one season. Live simply. That's the ticket. That's the '90s thing.

And then out of the corner came a great thumping sound. It was the bass line of of something that sounded like high-velocity disco. The corner exploded with swirling smoke and lights. We were all still nodding piously, but now, I happened to notice, we were nodding in time to the disco beat. Gradually, as a group, we began to reorient ourselves to the commotion in the corner and before I knew it, we were, as a group, walking towards the swirling fury of sound and light as if programmed from birth to do so. So much for '90s piety.

Just as we arrived, two young men came running down the runway and set to cutting, at top speed and with great flourishes, the hair of an understandably nervous brunette. They were dressed in black. Their hair fell in ringlets to their shoulders. They wore large bandannas across their foreheads. Voila! Hairdresser as rock-and-roll musician. This is, I have since discovered, a favourite look for certain stylists.

There is a single problem with these comparisons. Each tries to borrow the prestige of another profession. Under the circumstances, this is not a bad idea. Given the sheer hostility of the myths we have brought against hairdressers, how could it hurt? But claiming an affinity with other professions never seems, actually, to help. It has a nasty way of making hairdressing look worse, not better. Instead of adding prestige to hairdressing, it points out how little prestige there was in the first place. The hairdressing community always looks like it is trying too hard.

The medical comparison is especially dangerous. It provokes scepticism instead of admiration. Medicine is, after all, our highest-ranking profession. It is the exemplar of professional prestige. Anyone who dares compare himself to a doctor risks coming up short.

The comparison to art is also not a good idea. After all, artists have spent most of this century labouring to absent themselves from the contemporary world. Most of them have struggled to repudiate life in the real world, and they've done a pretty fine job of it. Hairdressers, by contrast, are creatures at the very heart of the contemporary world.

What's really annoying about these comparisons is that none of them captures the real character and importance of the hairdresser. None of them identifies the extraordinary transformational powers the good hairdresser has. And none acknowledges how important these powers make the hairdresser in the lives of his or her clients. In fact, for the process of self-transformation, hairdressers are at least as important as artists, rock stars and doctors.

Realities

So much for the falsehoods and the myths about hairdressing. Now it is time to turn to the realities. It is time for something a little more sophisticated. We need to replace the myths with a better, clearer view.

First, let's admit that these stereotypes are not completely fanciful. Perhaps hairdressers, consciously or unconsciously, live up to our expectations. We've all heard the stories. There are bad hairdressers in the world. There are hairdressers who live the stereotypes.

Some hairdressers secretly believe everything the stereotypes say about them

Laurie told the stylist [what] she wanted. According to her, he winced, then frowned. Finally he said: "You go to the doctor for an operation. You come here to be told how to wear your hair."[3]

These hairdressers like to have the upper hand. They like to keep clients waiting. They don't mind being rude or intimidating. They don't mind playing the bully. One hairdresser told me he deliberately intimidates his clients the moment they enter his salon.

I like to beat them up a bit. They need to know who they're dealing with. They need to know they need me more than I need them. It's kinda fun and kinda gross at the same time. I don't care. That's the way it is. Besides, it makes them [the clients] a lot easier to work with. Give them an inch. They'll take a mile.[4]

There are, I think, three reasons hairdressers end up living out the myth in this way. The first is the simple operation of supply and demand. As talented hairdressers begin to establish themselves, they find themselves in demand. And if they begin to rise from obscurity to local or national or even international fame, heads begin to swell. The best hairdressers must constantly fight the temptation to play the grandee.

But there is a darker reason. Some hairdressers secretly believe everything the stereotypes say about them. In their heart of hearts, they believe they are unimportant. An insecurity gnaws at them. The more they feel this insecurity, the more they swagger. Before long they are insufferable.

And darker still. Some hairdressers may be playing to our expectations, fulfilling the roles we've created for them. In this case, they are merely giving the client what she appears to demand. In this version, the client sustains the myth by demanding its performance every week at the salon.

For some hairdressers, however, it's simply pay-back time. For these professionals, there is something deeply galling about living in a society that refuses to recognize their worth. They can be at the top of their profession, the darling of hundreds of discerning clients, but as far as the rest of society is concerned, they're just simple-minded people doing a simple-minded job. Some hairdressers respond by putting on the ritz. You are going to refuse me my status? I will take it from you. Starved of recognition, they miss no opportunity to squeeze their clients for every bit of deference they can get. It's a simple game of status revenge.

There is an irony here, of course. When hairdressers act out this stereotype it costs them power. It's a simple equation. The less they listen, the less they can transform. The more they bully, the less they can engage. The more they intimidate, the less they can enlist. When they act like emperors, hairdressers trade the power of the magician for the crude and stupid satisfactions of a snob. And they give away what is their due: the ability to work with clients until hair and self change shape together.

Good hairdressers are another story altogether. Let's

return to the conversation between Cynthia and Bernard that appears at the beginning of this book. We can see here the myth-busting realities that pertain when a hairdresser really works with the client and begins to exercise the real powers of the profession. Let us set aside the stereotypes from inside and outside the world of hair and start again.

Ideals

Bernard opens the conversation by looking into the mirror, smiling and saying, "What's new, Cynthia?" This is a continuation of a series of ritual greetings that began from the moment he laid eyes on her and exclaimed: "Cynthia!" Good hairdressers follow the same rules for greeting that govern any greeting between friends. In both cases, the face expands with surprise and excitement: eyebrows flash upwards, mouth opens. The body follows suit: arms rise and outstretch, the body literally opens.

The psychological logic is clear enough: suffused with delight, the greeter opens emotionally to apprehend the other. And according to the sociological logic, the greeting sends a message: Take my delight as a measure of how much you mean to me. When Bernard "makes a fuss" over Cynthia, he is accomplishing the work of his profession. He is telling her that there is a connection between them, that she is "special" to him, that he prizes his connection to her.

Strictly speaking, greetings of this kind should not have much impact. After all, they are easy to counterfeit. We should not trust them. But we do. When friends and hairdressers react to the sight of us with these large and open gestures, we cannot help but feel a little pleased and a little honoured.

When you think about it, hairdressers are among the few parties to honour us this well or this dependably. Salespeople manufacture recognition and delight, but only for the duration of the sale. So do (some) people at work, but they tend to come and go. Apart from friends and relatives, who can be fickle, who but the hairdresser professes an unalloyed delight to see us on a routine, ongoing basis? The value of this recognition, especially in a society like our own, is very high. Almost no one else is really glad to see us.

The value of this ritual of recognition is primitive but powerful. Bernard's recognition allows Cynthia to say to herself, "I exist, I am approved, I am delightful, I am worthy." The character Al Franken created on "Saturday Night Live" ("I'm good enough, I'm smart enough and, gosh darn it, people like me") illustrates what life is like without this recognition; people denied it will supply their own.

A hairdresser like Bernard multiplies the effect with a *series* of recognitions. He remembers that Cynthia likes her coffee black and that she hates Milwaukee. He honours the hundred things he knows about her by never asking the wrong question or saying the wrong thing. Even before the haircut is complete, Cynthia begins to feel … better. There's something affirming about this place, it makes her feel welcome, approved, worthy. The rest of our world may be challenging, doubting, even mocking. Not Bernard. He offers her something like absolute and unconditional recognition.

Their two-minute conversation shows how hard Bernard is working at creating this impression. He is constantly working the conversation so that Cynthia remains at the centre of things. There are several moments at which Cynthia might ask about him, but she does not. She is content—nay, delighted—to have Bernard focus entirely on her.

There is an essential imbalance here. Bernard celebrates Cynthia with his greetings, his conversation, his solicitude. She reciprocates in only a vague sort of way. We have seen this kind of relationship before. It is the classic relationship that, in a sexist society, we construct between men and women. Traditionally, women suspend part of the self so that men can enjoy the luxuries of recognition. Traditionally, women give more emotional support to men than they get. Traditionally, they make sacrifices for which they are not fully compensated. What Bernard is doing for Cynthia is more typically (in a sexist society) what women do for men: suspending the self in the aggrandizement of the other.

The emotional consequences of this interaction are vast. Bernard creates for Cynthia an environment that is deeply affirming and deeply cossetting. Cynthia feels safe. She feels protected. And she begins to relax. This is part of the magic of the salon experience: that the client is so carefully attended to that she can begin to give up the protections and wariness that must otherwise be sustained. She can begin to unwind. She can start to space out. The terrible tight and protective wrapping that protects us from public scrutiny and attack is allowed to come undone. It's safe to come out. Cynthia does.

Bernard Becoming Cynthia Becoming Cynthia

So far we have treated Bernard as if he were a purely passive presence. We have made him sound like someone who merely honours the client. But the relationship goes deeper than this. Notice that Cynthia is in a bit of a lather about her relationship with her father. As it turns out, he's dating a woman Cynthia has not met, and this is awkward. On the one hand, Cynthia wonders whether she is not entitled to meet, and perhaps to vet, this woman. On the other, Cynthia accepts that a parent is entitled to go out with anyone he wants without seeking the approval of his child.

This anxiety has been circling in her mind for several days now and when she sits in Bernard's chair, it pops out. Bernard sizes up the problem immediately: Cynthia needs permission. He waits for his moment, and the next time she hesitates, he finishes the conversation assertively, clearly, definitively. He has literally put words in her mouth.

What Bernard is doing here is putting his self on loan. He takes Cynthia's part and says what she would like to say.

In this capacity, Bernard is not merely reflecting Cynthia. He is not merely shaping his self to her self. He is now actually *directing*. He is being clarifying and assertive. Now when he infuses Cynthia's self with his self, he becomes the hand within the puppet. He actually directs her to say what she cannot bring herself to say. Bernard helps Cynthia become Cynthia by becoming Cynthia himself.

Bernard as a Metamorph

Recall the bandage episode. Cynthia arrives wearing a bandage on her wrist. Bernard asks her what it is. Cynthia explains and says she has to keep herself from playing with the bandage. And Bernard at once begins to "play" with an imaginary bandage on his own hand. "Wow, is this ever neat!" And then again. "Hey, this is fun." Cynthia watches this with amusement. Bernard is now indulging himself in the very thing she has been trying not to do since she put the bandage on.

Bernard is always doing this. Cynthia talks about her boyfriend, her life at work, old school friends, her new dieting regime, her recent vacation to Arizona, the trip she's planning to Milan. All these things pour into Bernard, and he takes them in as part of his professionalism. There's a temptation to say here that Bernard is merely a "good listener," that he's a real "people person." Both of these are true, but the important point is that Bernard soaks up Cynthia's life in order to accomplish something extraordinary. He is putting himself at the disposal of the client in the most important way a hairdresser can. He is making himself a "parallel self."

The bandage example is a small one. Nothing astonishing happens when Bernard imagines aloud what it's like to play with a bandage. But this reflex, this willingness to become the client, happens over and over again in the relationship between the hairdresser and client. And this is the way hairdressers serve as metamorphs, as agents who transform themselves in order to transform the client.

Bernard the Monitor/Maker

Hairdressers tell me they are always listening for new events, important changes, new developments, anything that signals that a change is taking place in the client. This listening is necessary because the hairdresser needs to know what's next. Only thus can they help to prepare the client for what's to come.

One of the hairdressers I spoke to, Michael, offers a good example. He told me about a client who was headed for graduation from law school but still wearing her hair long and fly-away. Michael knew she could not take this look into the world of law, but the client did not know this. It was up to Michael to get her ready for the transition, not just in haircuts but in selves. He spent an entire year preparing her for the momentous cut, the one that would take her from her student days into professionalism.

Eventually, monster clients end up with a hairdresser too junior, too poor or too weak to resist their bullying

> By the time the day came, she was ready. I got her ready. We spent months talking about graduation and the new job. And I kept suggesting this cut and that cut. She wanted to keep her hair long but eventually she knew that she was going to have to go short. I broke her in slowly. And then the day came. We had a wake for her long hair the time before. And then, the next time, we went short.

Good hairdressers are a lot like flight instructors.

Clients: Myths, Realities and Ideals

Hairdressers delight in regaling one another with stories that demonstrate just how vain and peculiar the client can be. Clients are famous for flying off the handle at the least suggestion that they are not the centre of the universe.

Even the smallest thing can prove grounds for a temper tantrum: the hairdresser takes an incoming phone call, the hairdresser looks in on another client, or, that worst of all provocations, the coffee is not hot enough.

> These clients had huge egos. They were going to spend huge amounts of money and they wanted to make sure they got their rear ends kissed for every dollar.

In fact, this species of client is more rare than hairdressers would have you believe. But they do exist. And they are a nightmare. They expect to be pampered, indulged, forgiven, waited upon. They expect their wishes to be executed to the letter.

Vidal Sassoon tells a nice story about an imperial client in *Sorry I Kept You Waiting, Madam.* The client arrived in a Rolls Royce and entered the salon (Sassoon's first) with mink, chauffeur and Pekingese in tow. Sassoon began to work with her hair. He was interrupted.

> "One minute, young man," she said. "I haven't given you your instructions yet [which then were rattled off].... [Sassoon] swallowed and said gently, "But, madam—" [the client replied:] "But nothing. You heard me. Get on with it!"

It was, as Sassoon tells it, a moment of truth in the career of a young hairdresser. If he bowed to this woman, she would return, and so would her friends. If he resisted, he would lose a valued entrée into English society.

> As firmly as possible, I said, "I'm sorry, madam. We do not style hair that way here." For a moment she was silent, jowls heaving. Then she rasped, "Do as you're told!"[5]

Sassoon refused, and he lost the client. But not everyone can afford to treat rudeness this way. Every hairdresser is constantly having to contend with imperious clients, and even normally tranquil clients can have their moments.

Monster clients do exist. But the good news is that, normally, they get what they deserve: bad hairdressing. Eventually monster clients end up with a hairdresser too junior, too poor or too weak to resist their bullying. And then the trouble starts. The client has sealed herself away from the advice she needs to transform herself. Increasingly, she is locked into her own idea of what she should look like (for some reason, usually an enormous helmet of over-processed hair). Transformation stops. The self begins to drift further and further from the "now." Before long, the client has turned herself into a museum piece. This is the punishment for treating your hairdresser badly: self-parody.

Sam McKnight is the hairdresser for Princess Diana and Cindy Crawford. He knows what happens when people divorce themselves from a real relationship with their hairdresser.

> I think you're lucky if you know [on your own] when it's time to change. When you walk down the street and catch a glimpse of yourself in a window and say, "Oh my God, do I really look like that?" Well, you do, and you've got to start paying attention. When people don't change, they become caricatures of themselves.[6]

Realities

There are other ways the hairdresser-client relationship can break down. Take, for instance, the migrating client. These are clients who flit from hairdresser to hairdresser, never staying more than a couple of visits. Just when contact is being made, they move on.

Migrating clients are deeply irritating to hairdressers because they, too, make it impossible for real transformation to take place. They never let a hairdresser get to know them well enough to make a difference. They are constantly short-circuiting the relationship. As one hairdresser described it: "Everything you've invested in the relationship, everything you know about them, just walks out the door. This is not the way to cut hair."

One young woman, Jeannie, told me that when she decides "it's time for something new" she sets off in search of another hairdresser. In some sense, Jeannie knows exactly what she's doing. She does not want to commit herself to a single hairdresser because she does not want to fall within his influence or give up her autonomy. But the damage is clear. She has made it impossible for any hairdresser to supervise that crucial transition from cut to cut. Each new cut is being delivered by a perfect stranger.

There is also the "bad marriage" relationship. In this case, the client and hairdresser *do* have a long-term relationship with real interaction and consultation, but try as they might, they fail to establish a satisfactory working relationship. What they get instead are tense sessions, botched communications and bad haircuts.

Sometimes it's the hairdresser who is at fault. He isn't really listening. He never seems to "get" what's being said. The client comes away frustrated. "It's like we're always missing somehow," one client told me. There's no "somehow" about it. The hairdresser doesn't care. He doesn't believe clients know what they want. He simply does what he wants. The client is left looking at a new cut and thinking, "What does this have to do with what I asked for?"

> *I was surprised to discover how many women have been intimidated or antagonized by hairdressers*

But clients can also be at fault. They do not trust their hairdresser. They give him no real insight into the person they are or the person they are becoming. They starve him of essential information. And in the process they compromise him. The hairdresser is asked to supervise the client's transformation, but he is never in possession of the knowledge he needs to do so.

The relationship begins to feel like a marriage that's run out of gas. People are reduced to going through the motions. Genuine sympathy and regard have ceased. Neither party has the courage or the strength to put things right or to break things off. The relationship endures, but that is all it does. Between them, client and hairdresser manage to make their time together dreary and stultifying.

The Coming Revolt

The diplomatic difficulties between hairdresser and client are probably more serious than most hairdressers understand. My research suggests that there is something like a crisis looming in the industry. There are many clients who have simply opted out. They do not visit salons. They do not go to hairdressers. They cut their own hair or ask a friend to do it. They are simply out of the loop and show no evidence of wishing to return.

I was surprised to discover how many women have been intimidated or antagonized by hairdressers. These women have suffered so badly at the hands of incompetents that they are now in full flight. They have suffered bad colour, over-perming, uneven cuts and bad choices. They may never go back.

> One stylist gave me a perm and dyed my hair honey blond. It snapped off every time I touched it. The next guy gave me another perm "to make things right." Now I looked like I had red pubic hair on my head. Finally I went to the best stylist in town, and he sent me out looking like k.d. lang. It was three or four years before I let anyone touch a hair on my head.[7]

But these clients fear more than incompetence. They also fear the transformations the hairdresser will inflict upon them. They do not wish to relinquish control of their appearance to someone they see as meddling and troublesome.

I like styling it myself. I've had so much trouble going to hair salons. Usually they cut it okay, but I go in and tell them that I don't use a blow-drier or a curling iron, or mousse or hairspray. "No problem" they say, and the next thing you know they have the hairspray out. It's like, "Are you deaf? Didn't you hear what I just said?"

And then there are those who are in full revolt. These clients believe that if they relinquish control to a hairdresser, they are buying into the entire "beautification" industry. The moment they submit to the scissors, they lose control of their image and become dependent on the hairdresser. They make themselves complicit in an enterprise that defines women as objects and makes them second-class creatures. The moment they submit to the scissors, they surrender themselves to sexism.

You look beautiful when you leave the salon, just like the commercials say, and you go home and you try to do what they did and you can't do it. [Laughs] You end up with your hair standing up on end, and you look like an idiot. You can't wear a hat, and you can't go out in the wind. If you've got hairspray, it stays in the direction of the wind. It's just a nightmare.[8]

Hairdressers do create dependency. This was true, as we have seen, in the era of Antoine. Only the hairdresser could tease, spray, backcomb and sculpt the hair into its correct shape. Sassoon brought some liberation from this dependency by putting the shape of the hair in the cut of the hair, but even this did not eliminate dependency altogether. You still needed to have a hairdresser to keep your hair in trim. Sassoon was famous for demanding that his clients come into the salon several times a month to keep the cut perfect. Short styles require monthly visits, as do certain colour treatments. There is no way out of dependency except to break off the relationship altogether. And that's what some women have decided to do. They are "rebel angels" who have cast themselves out of the heavens of hairdressing.

Both these groups live quite happily outside the world of hairdressing. To be forced back on your own resources is *not* an option most women embrace with enthusiasm, but more and more women are absenting themselves from the conventional world of hair. A great defection is taking place. The client base is shrinking.

Ideals

This is the relationship in which hairdressers and clients work hand in glove. This is where they are linked by bonds of mutual respect, trust and affection. There are rocky moments from time to time, but the connection is deep and enduring.

How deep? It is not uncommon to hear hairdressers talk about clients as "family." Sometimes they feel closer to a woman than her own children. They even talk as if they have been "adopted" into the family.

> Oh yeah, we're family. She'd do anything for me. I'd do anything for her. She used to say when I moved she would fly the eight hundred miles to get her hair done. And I think she woulda, if I had let her. I'm her long lost son. I wouldn't be surprised if there was some connection in another life.

And the reverse is also true. Clients talk about hairdressers as long lost children, as the children they never had, or as children they wish they'd had instead. One matron told me:

> Harvey understands me … better than anyone … better than my kids, and much more than my husband. I sometimes wish Harvey could talk to them for me. I wish they knew me the way he does.

This closeness expresses itself in a hundred ways.

Hairdressers are invited to parties. They are sometimes invited to family events. Wealthy clients frequently lend their hairdressers winter condos and summer homes. Small talk adds up over the years. Lives intertwine. The hairdresser gets to see his client just before she goes to a big event, and he is there afterwards to hear about it in detail.

Normally, there are reciprocal privileges. The hairdresser lets his clients in on the joys and sorrows of his private life. And the client is always there in the chair to watch her hairdresser react as the events of the salon engage (and reveal) him. Thus do hairdresser and client make their way towards intimacy. Another transformation is taking place here: strangers become acquaintances, acquaintances become friends, friends become intimates.

There are clear distinctions between the lives of client and hairdresser. There are topics that are not talked about. There are boundaries over which people may not pass. And this is, generally, a good thing. There is nothing like a little privacy to get a relationship off the ground. This may seem paradoxical but, as Robert Frost observed, "Good fences make good neighbours." The last conversation you had with someone on a plane also makes the point.

One hairdresser told me that he is careful not to ask for too much or to see too much. "Do you ever feel like you are peering into people's souls?" I asked him.

> Oh sure. Clients will open up, especially when they're down. They will show you more than you can handle. There is definitely a confessional thing going on, sometimes, but I try to keep everything on the light side. You don't want them leaving more depressed than they came in.

The construction of intimacy is not, however, a purely mutual affair. It is the hairdresser who must be the initiating party. It is the hairdresser who negotiates the difficult waters of unfamiliarity and finds a way to friendship. Naturally, the client must be agreeable and forthcoming.

But if the relationship is a roaring success, most of the credit goes to the hairdresser. The great hairdresser, the real transformer, is gifted not just with the technical and artistic skills to execute great haircuts, he is also gifted with the extraordinary psychological skills necessary to fashion lives.

The toughest thing the hairdresser has to do is to involve the client. He must bring the client along until she, too, sees that the new shape is the necessary shape. He must create what one of my interviewees called "ownership."

> The client has to want the new cut as much as I do. They have to buy into it. They have to own it. Unless the client believes in the cut, they can't make it work. Then they come back to me and say, "Look what you've done to me."

The client needs enough "ownership" to take the chance on a new haircut and then keep her nerve through those opening days of uncertainty. She needs enough ownership to trust the hairdresser and the shape he is proposing. The worst-case scenario is when the client's nerve fails and she begins to repudiate both the cut and the cutter. Transformation breaks down. Hostilities begin to pool. Recriminations fly. The relationship falls apart.

So how is ownership created? The hairdresser must make the client a transformer too. He cannot simply make the decisions *de novo*, letting his client remain a passive party. After all, the client is the one who must enter the new look and live it. Unless she has helped create the look, she cannot inhabit it.

Establishing the Ideal Relationship

There is the possibility of perfection. This is where client and hairdresser fully achieve trust, intimacy and connection. It's where the hairdresser realizes the full power of his creativity and professionalism. It's where the client can begin self-invention on a new level. But it is not easy to get there. Clients and hairdressers must reinvent themselves to reinvent the relationship.

The first thing clients must do is to give up guilt. No more second thoughts. Time spent on hair and hairdresser is time well spent. It is a legitimate activity. (It is one of the really important things we do in our lives.) We are moving from one sense of self to another. One's hair is not a trivial matter. Talking to one's hairdresser is not a waste of time. Reading fashion magazines is not an indulgence. Hair care is self-invention. It's time to take it seriously. It's time to give up self-recrimination.

This second thing is for the client to get systematic. If hair care is self-invention, it's time to go about it in a more orderly way. It's time to do an inventory of where the client has been. What were the last five hairstyles? What aspects of the self did they succeed (or fail) to capture? And it's time to look ahead. What kind of self is now under construction?

The third thing the client can do is to establish a new relationship with her hairdresser. Good hairdressers can be superb partners in the process of self-transformation; bad hairdressers are worse than no help at all. If a hairdresser does not have the intelligence, sympathy and creativity to be a transformational partner, it's time to dump him. But it's important not to be too hasty. The client does not want to jettison her hairdresser until she has given him a fair try. She may need to become a new kind of client before he can become a new kind of hairdresser.

Clients should expect to spend more time and money on this relationship. They should expect to reveal more of themselves to their hairdressers. They are, after all, asking the hairdresser to build a parallel self inside himself, and he cannot do this without a richer, fuller relationship. To get more, the client must give more.

But in all of this the client must remember that she is the final arbiter of what happens. She is the one with the final say. Hers is the self that is under construction. She must learn to work well with her transformational partner, to give more to get more, but this must always be co-operation, not capitulation. Final authority rests with her.

Ideals: From the Hairdresser's Point of View

This is it. It's time for the hairdresser to leave the prison of stereotypes and slam the door behind him. Time to throw off all those stupid ideas about hairdressers being flighty, irresponsible, insubstantial and dim.

And this is the time for hairdressers to throw off their own stereotypes. Forget the comparisons to doctors, priests, rock stars. In crucial ways, hairdressers are just as important. They are the professionals who stand at the transformational heart of the contemporary world. They are the new high priests of self-definition.

Historically, the time is right. No other profession has as legitimate a claim to the role of the metamorph. No existing profession can perform this service quite as the hairdresser does. Hairdressers are our transformers. It is they who advise women as they make their way from one self to another. The time is right for them to seize the opportunity, to make themselves the metamorphic profession.

But it won't be easy. If they wish to be the new profession in charge of transformation, hairdressers must reinvent themselves. Too many crucial decisions are being made in haste at the chair under the pressure of a deadline, an impatient client and a noisy salon. New responsibilities demand new methods.

It is necessary to take more time with clients. It is necessary to do periodic consultations, off the floor, away from the cutting and colouring. Client and hairdresser must meet face to face and talk. It is necessary to keep a written and a Polaroid record of the good cuts and the bad ones. It is necessary to rehearse the client's options to a client in a more systematic way; style books will not do it any more. It is necessary to get to know the client, to listen to her, with more and better care. It is necessary to take the file home at night and dwell on where a client should be headed.

And here's the bad news. Hairdressers will have to charge more. Adding value to the relationship will have to add costs. More to the point, as metamorphs, hairdressers deserve to get paid for the crucial service they are rendering. The good ones are given an enormous responsibility. They accomplish an enormous private good. They deserve to be paid accordingly.

Hair: The Shape of Things to Come

We know that transformation will be one of the important themes of the twenty-first century. Everything points in this direction. Already we live in a world that teems with change. Some of it—the plastic surgery, the weight-lifting, the skipping from self to self—is intentional. Some of it is a forced response to the continual variety, experiment and restlessness of our society. Active or reactive, change is now the order of the day, the brute fact of our private and public lives.

Furthermore, we know that the twenty-first century will usher in new transformational technologies. Computer technologies are on the verge of manipulating meaning beyond anything ever dreamed of by the masters of moveable type and the conventional rhetorics of art and literature. You don't need to be Marshall McLuhan to see these will change the very nature of our perception and experience.

But these computer technologies will be nothing compared to the inventions of biotechnology. Suddenly we will be able to transform the very stuff of our physical existence. We will eventually be able to work and rework any aspect of this thing we call the body. Once we wave this Ovid's wand, there is no telling where we will end up. All we can say for certain is that, in the long term, this technology will transform us beyond recognition.

Do we have a template for any of this? Do we have a

way of guessing what we will do with the new computer and biological technologies of the next century? Do we have anything in our present experience of the world that can give us a glimpse of what lies ahead?

I think we do. We can begin by taking hair seriously.

This is one of our best indications of how we will use these technologies to reinvent ourselves. Hair provides a splendid chance to glimpse what a fully metamorphic world will feel like. It may be our best chance to prepare for the cataclysmic changes that await us.

The second question is just as pressing: Who now controls this knowledge? The answer will not sit well in Washington, for this metamorphic technology is the domain of two unlikely groups: women and hairdressers. Both are practised and cunning in a way that men and other professions cannot begin to be. These two groups have, as it were, the home field advantage. They know how to do what we will all have to do. They are ready for the next century while the rest of us are not.

Ironically, both groups have been made to pay hugely for their mastery of hair. Women and hairdressers have been damned as light-headed, trivial, superficial for their trouble. We have heaped contempt and ridicule on them and cast doubt on their intelligence, morality and seriousness.

It is time for these two groups to step forward and claim their due. And they might as well do so together. It is working in tandem, in the perfect partnership of the really good hairdresser-client relationship, that these two parties can seize the opportunity before them. It is by transcending the myths and the falsehoods that they can seize the time.

Will hairdressers and clients take up the challenge? Will they transform their relationship to instruct the world in the arts of self-transformation? We shall have to wait and see. Historically, the moment is perfect. We have seen Bernard and Cynthia working on it in an unofficial way. The question is whether they will share it with the rest of us.

Endnotes

Chapter One
1. Naomi Wolf (1991), *The Beauty Myth: how images of beauty are used against women* (New York: William Morrow and Co., Inc.). See also Wendy Chapkis (1986), *Beauty Secrets* (Boston: South End Press) and Kathrin Perutz (1970), *Beyond the Looking Glass: Life in the beauty culture* (Middlesex: Penguin).

Chapter Two
1. Holly Brubach (1992), "In Fashion: Sackcloth and Ashes," *The New Yorker*, LXVII (50 February 3), 78-82, p. 78.

Chapter Three
1. Ruth Murrin (1955), "Spray to Make Your Hair Behave," *Good Housekeeping*, 141 (2 August), 125–126.
2. In Anon. (1971), "Men In Vogue," *Vogue* (British edition), 128 (1 January), 19.
3. Grant McCracken (n.d.), "Cars in Space: Progress, Science, Technology, Gender and Flight motifs in the 1950s American Automobile," manuscript in progress.
4. These notes on Adler and the quotes contained in it come from Maurice Zolotow (1958), "Hairdresser to the stars," *Saturday Evening Post*, 231 (13 September 23), pp. 32–33, 96–98.
5. Most of this account of Alexandre comes from an illuminating piece by Katharine Whitehorn (1963), "Alexandre the Great," *Ladies' Home Journal*, 80 (9 December), pp. 148–153.
6. Grant McCracken (1988), "The Making of Modern Consumption," ch. 2 of *Culture and Consumption* (Bloomington: Indiana University Press).

7. Linda MacNish (1967), "The changing hairdos of Princess Margaret," *Good Housekeeping*, 164 (1 January), pp. 30–31.

8. Rosemary Blackmon (1962), "World's Greatest Hairdressers," *Vogue*, 140 (7 October 15), pp. 99–104, 162.

9. This account stems mostly from Ernest O. Hauser (1956), "He Domineers Beautiful Women," *Saturday Evening Post*, 229 (12), 28–29, 109–113.

Chapter Four

1. In Judy Klemesrud (1966), "Sassoon refuses to finger-wave for state test," *New York Times* (September 20), p. 51.

2. Recorded by Priscilla Tucker, New York *Herald Tribune*, quoted in Vidal Sassoon (1968), *Sorry I Kept You Waiting, Madam* (New York: G.P. Putnam's Sons), p. 195.

3. In Judy Klemesrud (1966), "Sassoon refuses to finger-wave for state test," *New York Times* (September 20), p. 51.

4. Susanne Kirtland (1963), "The Revolt Against Fancy Hairdos," *Look*, 27 (14 July), p. 37.

5. Eleanor Haris (1963), "Overteased Hair," *Look*, 27 (14 July), pp. 26-32.

6. Anon. (1962), "Real Regal," *Newsweek*, March 12, 1962, p. 92.

7. Vidal Sassoon (1968), *Sorry I Kept You Waiting, Madam* (New York: G.P. Putnam's Sons), p. 77.

8. Diane Fishman and Marcia Powell (1993), *Vidal Sassoon: Fifty Years Ahead* (New York: Rizzoli International Publications).

9. In Gerald Battle-Welch, Luca P. Marighetti and Werner Moller (1992), *Vidal Sassoon und das Bauhaus* (Edition Cantz), pp. 7-10, p. 8.

10. Vidal Sassoon (1968), *Sorry I Kept You Waiting, Madam* (New York: G.P. Putnam's Sons), p. 178. Sassoon's formulation raises the question that Peter Laslett at Cambridge has long bid us ask: Just why was it that England was the birthplace of the industrial and consumer revolutions?

11. Eric Fridman, "Haircut," *American Scholar*, v. 60, Summer 1991, p. 433.

Chapter Five

1. Rita Freedman (1986), *Beauty Bound* (Lexington: D.C. Heath and Company), p. 196; Patricia Schultz (1991), "All American Blondes," *Harper's Bazaar*, February, 154-157; Anthony Synnott, "Shame and Glory: a sociology of hair," *British Journal of Sociology*, XXXVIII (3), 381-413, p. 388.

2. Recorded in Toronto on June 5, 1991. Speakers were members of a large public sector organization: a female secretary (with red hair) and a female administrative assistant (blond).

3. Freda Garmaise (1987), "Brazen Blonde," *Ms. Magazine* (November), pp. 30-34, p. 30.

4. Paul Rudnick (1990), "Talking Fashion: Platinum is Preferred," *Vogue* (January), pp. 230-232.

5. Grant McCracken (1988), "Ever Dearer in Our Thoughts: Patina and the representation of status before and after the eighteenth century," pp. 31-43 in *Culture and Consumption* (Bloomington: Indiana University Press).

6. Gloria Steinem (1988), *Marilyn: Norma Jean* (New York: Signet), p. 206.

7. Steinem, *Marilyn: Norma Jean*, p. 206.

8. This account of Marilyn Monroe rests mostly on the work of Steinem and Mailer. My particular debts to them are acknowledged throughout these footnotes. I have also examined (and recommend) two fundamental treatments: Fred Lawrence Guiles (1984), *Legend, the Life and Death of Marilyn Monroe* (New York: Stein and Day) and Maurice Zolotow (1960), *Marilyn Monroe* (New York: Harcourt, Brace and Jovanovich).

9. In Steinem, *Marilyn: Norma Jean*, pp. 47-48.

10. In Norman Mailer (1973), *Marilyn: a biography* (New York: Grosset and Dunlap), p. 68.

11. In Steinem, *Marilyn: Norma Jean*, pp. 90.

12. Anon. (1941), "Veronica Lake's Hair: It is a cinema property of world influence," *Life*, 11 (21), pp. 58-61.

13. George Eells, and Stanley Musgrove (1982), *Mae West: A biography* (New York: William Morrow and Company), p. 26.

14. Molly Haskell (1974, reprint 1987), *From Reverence To Rape: the Treatment of Women in the Movies* (Chicago: University of Chicago Press), p. 113, 114.

15. "By 1952, Marilyn had graduated to stardom and the quintessential dumb blond—Lorelei Lee in *Gentlemen Prefer Blondes* ..." Steinem, *Marilyn: Norma Jean*, p. 96.

16. Mailer, *Marilyn: a biography*, p. 15.

17. In Anon. (1990), "Cutting edge model Linda Evangelista drops a blond bombshell on the fashion world, color it disapproving," *People*, 34 (20 November 19, 1990), p. 178.

18. In Tom Fennell (1991), "The Best in the World," *Maclean's* 104 (49 Dec. 9, 1991), pp. 36-40.

19. In David Livingstone (1992), "Model Behavior," *Saturday Night*, 107 (2 March), pp. 36-76.

20. In Livingstone, "Model Behavior," *Saturday Night*, pp. 36-76.

21. Camille Paglia (1992), "Madonna II: Venus of the Radio Waves," in *Sex, Art and American Culture* (New York: Random House), p. 10.

22. Camille Paglia (1992), "Madonna I: Animality and Artifice," in *Sex, Art and American Culture*, p. 4.

Chapter Six

1. L. Logan (1992), "The Brunette Majority," *Mademoiselle*, 97 (February), pp. 104–107, p. 106.

2. In Stanley Frank (1961), "Brunette Today, Blonde Tomorrow," *Saturday Evening Post*, 234 (36), pp. 20-21, 45-46, p. 46.

3. Anon. (1990), *Vogue* (February), p. 314.

4. E. Collier (1991), "Bold Brunette," *Glamour*, 89 (August), p. 193.

5. Logan, "The Brunette Majority," *Mademoiselle*, pp. 104-107.

6. E. Collier (1991), "Bold Brunette," *Glamour*, 89 (August), p. 193.

7. Georgia Dullea (1992), "Head of the Class," *New York Times*, 60 (May 31, 1992), section 5, p. 1.

8. Laura Flynn McCarthy (1990), "Images: hair answers," *Vogue* 180 (July), p. 86.

9. McCarthy, "Images: hair answers," *Vogue*, p. 86.

10. Deborah Grace Winer (1988), "The Redhead Revealed," *Seventeen*, 47 (3 March), 246-247, 275-276, p. 276.

11. Carol Krucoff (1983), "The Rise of Redhead Power," *Psychology Today*, 17 (February), p. 18.

12. Saul Feinman and George W. Gill (1978), "Sex differences in physical attractiveness preferences," *The Journal of Social Psychology*, 105 (June), 43-52, p. 50.

13. Dennis E. Clayson and Michael L. Klassen (1989), "Perception of Attractiveness by Obesity and Hair Color," *Perceptual and Motor Skills*, 68 (1 February), 199-202, p. 199.

14. Dennis E. Clayson and Micol R. C. Maughan (1986), "Redheads and Blonds, Stereotypic Images," *Psychological Reports*, 59 (2 October), 811-816.

15. Winer, "The Redhead Revealed," *Seventeen*, p. 276.

16. Krucoff, "The Rise of Redhead Power," *Psychology Today*, p. 18.

17. This treatment of redheaded children is apparently routine in our culture. Pennebaker says her redheaded child is routinely treated like a "movie star." Ruth Pennebaker (1990), "Raising a Redhead," *Parents*, 65 (11 November), 106-108, p. 108.

18. Tom Robbins (1988), "Ode to Redheads," *Gentleman's Quarterly*, 58 (June), 216-219.

19. Hairdresser in Toronto, interviewed September 1991.

20. In Winer, "The Redhead Revealed," *Seventeen*, p. 276.

21. Anon. (1987), "Reds turn on the heat," *Harper's Bazaar*, 120 (July), 108-111.

22. Sally Riddles (1987), "Your Redhead Beauty Guide," *Harper's Bazaar*, 120 (July), 108, 109, 157, 158, p. 109.

23. Linda Wells (1988), "Red is right now," *New York Times Magazine*, Aug. 7, 1988, pp. 52-53.

24. Colleen Sullivan (1989), "Images: Hair," *Vogue*, 179 (October), p. 212, 218.

25. Riddles, "Your Redhead Beauty Guide," *Harper's Bazaar*, p. 109.

26. All quotes for Georgette Mosbacher and the biographical details of this section are taken from James Servin (1992), "One Tough Redhead," *Allure*, 2 (8 August), 68.

27. For more on Hayworth's transformation, see pp. 146-153 in Otto Friedrich (1986), *City of Nets: A Portrait of Hollywood in the 1940's* (New York: Harper and Row, Publishers).

28. Friedrich, *City of Nets: A Portrait of Hollywood in the 1940's*, p. 269.

Chapter Seven

1. In Stanley Frank (1961), "Brunette Today, Blonde Tomorrow," *Saturday Evening Post*, 234 (36), pp. 20-21, 45-46, p. 46. This remark now offends our sensibilities on both racist and sexist counts. It is likely that there was however a method to Revson's madness. He objected to the use of bleach because his company did not support "do it yourself" dye jobs and sold only to salons.

2. In Frank, "Brunette Today, Blonde Tomorrow," *Saturday Evening Post*, pp. 20-21, 45-46, p. 46.

3. In Frank, "Brunette Today, Blonde Tomorrow," *Saturday Evening Post*, pp. 20-21, 45-46, p. 45.

4. Anon. (1950), "This lady is dyeing her hair," *Life*, 29 (22, November 27), pp. 113, 115-116, p. 113.

5. Anon. (1951), "Powdered Streaks," *Life*, 32 (20, May 19), pp. 101-102. The concern for the healthiness of hair dyeing has not gone away. In M. Parker (1992), "Dyeing May Be Hazardous to Your Health," *Newsweek*, 120 (12, July 13), p. 59, new and disturbing evidence is recounted.

6. Anon. (1953), "Quite a piece of change: $90,000,000 spent last year for hair colourings," *Vogue* (January 1), pp. 138-139, p. 139.

7. Anon. (1957), "What color hair do you want?" *Look*, 21 (23), pp. 76-79, p. 77.

8. In Frank, "Brunette Today, Blonde Tomorrow," *Saturday Evening Post*, pp. 20-21, 45-46, p. 45.

9. Anon. (1962), "Airlines: Hair pulling," *Newsweek*, 59 (24, June 11), p. 77.

10. Anon. (1963), "Color Me Anything," *Newsweek*, 62 (8, August 19), p. 55.

11. Anon. (1991), "Color comes on strong," *Vogue* (February), pp. 325-326.

12. Georgia Dullea (1981), "Do Grays Have More Fun? Just Ask Them," *New York Times* (March 1), p. 55.

13. Anon. (1988), "Haircolor: the new realities," *Vogue* (September), p. 281-282, p. 281.

14. J. Sirob (1992), "Hair to dye for," *Working Woman*, 17 (January), pp. 70, 72, 87, p. 72.

15. Anon. (1991), "Color comes on strong," *Vogue* (February), p. 325-326, p. 326.

16. H.L. Schifter (1991), "Haircolor art," *Harper's Bazaar*, 124 (October 3358), pp. 44, 48, 52, 54, p. 52.

17. Schifter, "Haircolor art" *Harper's Bazaar* (October 3358), pp. 44, 48, 52, 54.

18. In Marcia Menter (1992), "Is your hair aging too fast?" *Redbook*, 178, (5), pp. 52, 54, 58.

19. *The Concise Columbia Dictionary of Quotations* (New York: Columbia University Press, 1989).

20. Kathryn Hughes (1993), "Some People are Dyeing to Go Grey," *Globe and Mail*, August 24, 1993, p. A18.

21. Anna Qindlen (1991), "Point of View: Going Grey," *Redbook*, 177 (6 October), pp. 21-22, p. 21.

22. Dullea, "Do Grays Have More Fun? Just Ask Them," *New York Times*, p. 55.

23. Dullea, "Do Grays Have More Fun? Just Ask Them," *New York Times*, p. 55.

Chapter Eight

1. Sarah Lyall (1992), "Big hair is rearing its head at the malls," *New York Times*, March 4, p. C1.

2. Gail Huitt in Kevin Helliker (1991), "Hair is big in Dallas, and that troubles Roger Thompson," *Wall Street Journal*, January 29, p. 1, 12; and personal communication. "Rat" means "tease" and "tar" means, roughly, "hell."

3. Details and quote from Helliker, "Hair is big in Dallas and that troubles Roger Thompson," *Wall Street Journal*, p. 1, 12; and personal communication with Mr. Thompson.

4. Lyall, "Big hair is rearing its head at the malls," *New York Times*, pp. C1, C6, p. C6.

5. Aileen Ribeiro (1978), "The Macaronis," *History Today*, 7, 463-468.

6. Georgine deCourtais (1973), *Women's Headdress and Hairstyles*, (London: B.T. Batsford), p. 80.

7. Thorstein Veblen (1899/1912), *The Theory of the Leisure Class* (New York: Macmillan).

8. Richard Corson (1965), *Fashions in Hair: The First Five Thousand Years* (London: Peter Owen), p. 394.

9. Mary Burt Baldwin (1962), "Teen-age girls show decided preference for Bouffant hairdos," *New York Times*, February 24, p. 20.

10. M. Fromow (1965), "Frou frou curls," *Good Housekeeping*, 161 (6, December), pp. 92-95.

11. Anon. (1960), "The guiche: not a dance or a dish, it's the newest French curl," *Life*, 49 (24, December 12), pp. 61-62, 67-68.

12. Mary Burt Baldwin (1962), "Teen-age girls show decided preference for Bouffant hairdos," *New York Times*, February 24, p. 20.

13. Kathleen Deveny (1993), "The Decline of Big Hair," *Wall Street Journal*, September 13, p. B1.

14. M. Murphy, "Brenda's imitators: Cutting their hair just like mine ..." *T.V. Guide*, 39 (34 August 24), pp. 8-12.

15. M. Gravenas (1992), 'Our love/hate affair with hair," *Glamour*, 90 (October), pp. 222-229, p. 228.

16. Claire Scovell (1991), "Long Hair Really is Sexier," *Cosmopolitan*, 211 (5, November), p. 56.

17. Anon. (1990), "Hair Power: Long, Wild, Tumultuous Looks Make the Best-Tressed List," *Harper's Bazaar*, February, pp. 150-153, p. 150.

18. As quoted in James H. McAlexander and John W. Schouten (1989), "Hair Style Changes as Transition Markers," *Sociology and Social Research*, 74 (1 October), pp. 58-62.

19. Sally Wadyka (1993), "New Girls in Town," *Mademoiselle*, 99 (3 March), p. 195.

20. Monica M. Moore and Diana L. Butler (1989), "Predictive Aspects of Nonverbal Courtship Behavior in Women," *Semiotica*, 76(3-4): 205-215.

21. Euripides (1988), *The Bacchae*, in *Euripides, Plays: One*, J. Michael Walton, trans. (London: Methuen), p. 118.

22. John Aubrey (1987), *Aubrey's Brief Lives*, Oliver Lawson Dick, ed. (London: Penguin Books), p. 100.

23. Elisabeth G. Gitter (1984), "The Power of Women's Hair in

the Victorian Imagination," *PMLA*, 99 (5 October), pp. 936-954, p. 938.

24. Anon. (1941), "Veronica Lake's hair is a cinema property of world influence," *Life*, 11 (21), pp. 58-61.

25. Anon. (1965), "All Ironed Out," *Newsweek*, 65 (1 January 11), p. 53.

26. Patricia Peterson (1964), "Let it Fall," *New York Times Magazine* (May), p. 48+.

27. Carrie Donovan (1991), "By Design: new twists in hairdos," *New York Times*, December 10, B18; see also Carrie Donovan (1991), "By Design: Hair; Wear it Long and Loose," *New York Times* (April 16), B6.

28. S. Tuck (1991), "Right hair, right now," *Rolling Stone*, November 28, pp. 79-80, 82.

29. Peter York (1980), "New Model," *Style Wars* (London: Sidgwick and Jackson), pp. 87-94.

30. Anon. (1977), "Who's the Farrahest?" *Newsweek*, 89 (26, June 27), p. 58.

31. Roger Rosenblatt (1977), "The back of the book: don't change a hair for me," *New Republic*, 176 (9, February 26), pp. 29-30.

32. In Anon. (1978), "Summer Hairlines," *Vogue* (British ed.), 135 (8, June), pp. 142-143.

33. Karl E. Meyer (1977), "The Barbie Doll as Sex Symbol," *Saturday Review*, 5 (1, October 1), p. 45.

34. Blair Sabol (1977), "Far-r-out fitness … Farrah's way," *Vogue*, 167 (4, April), pp. 128-129.

35. Lois Long (1954), "The Shaggy Hair Story," *The New York Times Magazine*, May 30, pp. 18-19, 32.

36. Madge Garland, *The Changing Face of Beauty* (London: Weidenfeld and Nicolson), p. 205.

37. I owe this suggestion to Susan Pointe.

38. Richard Corson (1965), *Fashions in Hair, the First Five Thousand Years* (London: Peter Owen), p. 361.

39. Anon. (1955), "Precious Parisienne," *Life*, 38 (20, May 16), pp. 94-102, p. 94.

40. Anon. (1955), "Arriving in Manhattan…," *Time*, 65 (17, April 25), p. 41.

41. In Paul D. Zimmerman (1967), "Twiggy in America," *Newsweek*, 69 (15, April 10), pp. 62-66, p. 65.

42. Vidal Sassoon (1968), *Sorry I Kept You Waiting, Madam* (New York: G.P. Putnam's Sons), p. 14.

43. Notice the dates of these articles: "the fashion for 1961 will be short hair," in Milton Bracker 1960. "Girls to Get Curls in '61,

Paris Hears," *New York Times*, Nov. 14, p. 41; "The big trend is toward short hair," Alexandre, quoted in Charlotte Cutis, 1962. "Coiffeur Here 'to Make a Revolution,'" *New York Times*, October 11; Angela Taylor, 1972, "Pendulum Swings Back to Short Hair," *New York Times*, CXXI (14,837, Aug. 10), p. 31; Anon., 1973, "Summer Shortcut," *Time*, 102 (3, July 16), pp. 58-59; Anon., 1982, "Hair Cut Short," *New York Times Magazine*, September 26, p. 84; Camille Cozzone, 1991, "Short Circuit," *Harper's Bazaar*, April, pp. 26, 28; Lindsy Van Gelder, 1993, "Beyond Big Hair: Getting Sick of Long Hair? You're in Good Company," *Allure* (3, 3 March), pp. 124-7.

44. In Camille Cozzone (1991), "Short Circuit," *Harper's Bazaar*, April, pp. 26, 28, p. 28.

45. Tina Gaudoin (1994), "The Devil Made Me Do It," *New York Times Magazine*, Part 2, Spring, pp. 22-32, p. 32.

46. Ronny H. Cohen (1979), "Tut and the '20s: The 'Egyptian Look,'" *Art in America*, 67 (2), p. 97.

47. Corson, *Fashions in Hair, the First Five Thousand Years*, pp. 606-619. See also F. Scott Fitzgerald (1920, 1989), "Bernice Bobs Her Hair," in *The Short Stories of F. Scott Fitzgerald*, Matthew J. Bruccoli, ed. (New York, Charles Scribner's Sons), pp. 24-47.

48. R.P. Weston and Bert Lee (1926), "Shall I Have It Bobbed Or Shingled" (Toronto: Leo Feist Limited).

49. Marcel Haedrich (1971, reprint 1972), *Coco Chanel, Her Life, Her Secrets* (Boston: Little, Brown and Co.), p. 120.

50. Charlotte Curtis (1962) "The Movies Are Staging Comeback as Influence on Fashion and Hairdos," *New York Times*, July 13, p. 26.

51. Dylan Jones (1990), *Haircuts: Fifty Years of Styles and Cuts* (London: Thames and Hudson).

52. Angela Taylor (1969), "Page Boy Never Died," *New York Times*, March 18, p. 48.

53. Anon. (1991), "Personal Style: Cut," *McCall's*, 119 (1 October), p. 72.

54. Anon. (1954), "Which Hair Style?" *Life* 36 (7, February 15), pp. 67-70. See also Anon. (1953), "Nibble at the Neck," *Life* 35, (2), pp. 93-96.

55. Anon. (1958), "A New Look in American Fashion Based On Hair," *Vogue*, 131 (3 February), pp. 108-109, p. 108.

56. Anon., "Suzy Parker has her first haircut," *Vogue* 145 (June), pp. 118-121.

57. Elizabeth Collier, "Curls are making a comeback," *Vogue*, 180 (November), p. 224.

58. In Rowann Gillman (1990), "The One Inch Solution,"

Working Woman (15, September), pp. 190-192, p. 192.

59. Jones, *Haircuts: Fifty Years of Styles and Cuts*, p. 87.

60. Jones, *Haircuts: Fifty Years of Styles and Cuts*, p. 7.

61. Anon. (1954), "Feminine Butch: Summer Cut is Shortest Yet," *Life* (37, 3, July 19), pp. 68-70.

62. In Anon. (1964), "His and Hers," Life and Leisure Section, *Newsweek*, 64 (6 August 10), p. 64. See also Gloria Emerson (1964), "Esterel to Shave Models' Heads for Fall Show," *New York Times*, July 3, 1964, p. 24.

63. In Steve Dougherty (1988), "Sinead O'Connor. A Poetic Irish Popstar with a Hit Record and Very Little Hair," *People*, 29 (19), pp. 146-147, p. 146.

64. Gloria Emerson (1969), "British Youth's Latest Turn: The Skinhead," *The New York Times*, Dec. 16, p. 12.

65. Richard Sandomir (1993), "Beyond the Fringe: The Boldly Bald," *New York Times*, May 5, p. C1.

Chapter Nine

1. Jay Scott (1990), "Designer Death," pp. 9-13 in Cary Fagan and Robert MacDonald, eds., *Streets of Attitude* (Toronto: Yonge and Bloor).

2. Anon. (1965), "Customs: Keeping the Hair Up," *Time*, 86 (27 December 31, 1965), p. 28.

3. In Bob Levey (1991), "At the Salon: Arrogance, Not Elegance." *The Washington Post*, November 28, p. E1.

4. From an interview conducted in New York City, fall of 1992.

5. Vidal Sassoon (1968), *Sorry I Kept You Waiting, Madam* (New York: G.P. Putnam's Sons), pp. 83-84.

6. Quoted in Kathy Healy (1992), "Behind the Scenes With a Virtuoso Stylist," *Allure*, 2 (September 9), 136-141, p. 140.

7. Louise Lague (1990), "Hairstyles from hell," *Glamour*, 88 (August), pp. 198-192.

8. Interview conducted in Toronto in January 1993.

Photo credits

Every effort has been made to contact or trace all copyright holders. The publisher will be pleased to make good any errors or omissions brought to our attention in future editions.

Courtesy: Styles on Video: page 5.
CPS: pages 11, 21, 26, 28, 29, 35, 36, 64, 68, 69 (both), 72, 73, 75, 76, 77, 78, 81, 82, 85, 89, 91, 93, 96, 97, 98, 101, 108, 109, 119, 128, 133, 134, 139, 140, 141, 144, 145, 149, 152, 153, 157, 161, 163, 169, 171, 176, 177 and 178.
Photographer, Dare Wright: page 31.
Judy Nisenholt, Photography: pages 33, 34 and 129.
Museum of Cosmetology Arts & Sciences: pages 38, 113 (both) and 158.
Photographer, Hans Knopf: page 39.
Photographer, John Launois: page 41.
Baron, CPS: page 42.
Authenticated News Photo, Culver pictures Inc.: page 44.
Ted Knowles—Vogue Studio: page 45.
Photographer, David Montgomery: page 47.
Photographer, Roger Thompson: page 53 (top).
Photographer, Terence Donovan: page 53 (bottom).
Photographer, David Bailey: page 54.
Mark VanManen, *The Vancouver Sun*, CPS: page 58 and 181.

Photo by Barry Lategan: page 61.
Ladies Home Journal, CPS: page 66.
ABC Ajansi, CPS: page 67.
Reed Saxon, CPS: page 71.
B. Spremo/*Toronto Star*, CPS: page 86 and 159.
Wyatt Counts, CPS: page 94.
Ron Edwards, CPS: page 100.
R. La Blanc, CPS: page 105.
T. Wood, CPS: page 106.
Gilbert Tourte, CPS: page 118.
Bob Daugherty, CPS: page 121.
Drew, CPS: page 124.
Bernard Brault, CPS: page 127.
Colonial Williamsburg Foundation: page 131.
L. Cironneau, CPS: page 135.
Cover art © 1993 Harlequin Enterprises Limited. Reprinted
with permission: page 137.
Marty Lederhander, CPS: page 147.
Bettmann Archives: page 155.
Martin Keene, CPS: page 172.

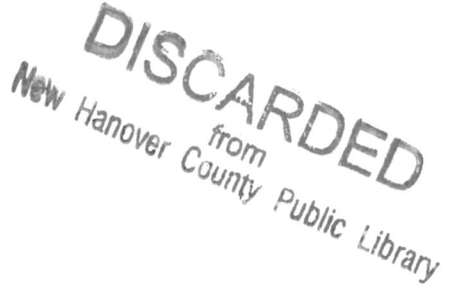